DON'T LET YOUR

HORMONES

RUIN YOUR LIFE

Dr Sandra Cabot, M.B.B.S.,D.R.C.O.G., is a well known media doctor and author of the best selling book *Women's Health* and also *Menopause — You Can Give It A Miss!*

Sandra is a consultant to the Australian Women's Health Advisory Service, has regularly appeared on many national TV shows, including the Ray Martin Midday Show, had her own talk back show on radio 2GB for two years, writes for *Woman's Day* magazine and is a much sought after public speaker on women's health. She has extensive clinical experience in women's health, hormonal disorders and naturopathic medicine.

Sandra is sometimes known as the 'flying doctor' as she frequently flies herself to many of Australia's country towns to hold health forums for rural women. These help to raise funds for local women's refuges and women's health services. She spent considerable time working in the Department of Obstetrics and Gynaecology in a large missionary hospital in the Himalayan foothills of India.

Sandra has communicated with women via TV and radio and receives thousands of letters from women all over Australia. Thus she is acutely aware of the health problems and needs of women from many different backgrounds.

First published in 1991 by Women's Health Advisory Service
155 Eagle Creek Rd, Werombi, NSW 2570. (046) 531 445
Reprinted 1991, 1993, 1994 (twice)

Cabot, Sandra
  Don't let your hormones ruin your life says Dr Sandra Cabot
  Bibliography
  Includes index

  ISBN 0 646 04935 6

  1. Hormones — Physiological effect. 2. Women — Health and
  hygiene. 3. Postpartum depression — Treatment.
  4. Premenstrual syndrome.
  I. Women's Health Advisory Service (NSW) II. Title

Printed and bound in Australia by
Australian Print Group, Melbourne Australia

CONTENTS

ACKNOWLEDGEMENTS

I would like to acknowledge the professional
skills of my two editors and dear friends, Diane
Blackwell and Stephanie Lewis who helped me
to put the very complicated and technical
subject of endocrinology into a format that
every woman can understand.
I would also like to thank Lydia Sharan who
transcribed my thoughts and voice into words
with her computer and typing skills.

FOREWORD

by Dr Oscar Horky M.B., B.S., F.R.C.O.G., D.G.O. (Paris), F.R.A.C.O.G.

I have followed Dr Sandra Cabot's medical progress over the last 15 years with great interest, and increasing admiration. Her understanding of human beings and their ills was apparent from her earliest days in practice. It was my pleasure to be involved in mutually treating patients, and to observe her dealing first hand with the sick. She developed a technique of healing the whole person, and not just one organ.

Dr Cabot uses the total pharmacopoeia and has proven that modern medicine can and must co-exist with naturopathic therapies. Needless to say, her fame spread to such a degree that she could not possibly attend to all who needed her. A lesser person would have left it at that, but not Dr Cabot. For those she could not personally see, she wrote a book, *Women's Health* and then another, *Menopause — You Can Give It A Miss!* and now another.

This latest one deals with the most intricate and complex of all medical subjects: hormones and the endocrine system. A scholarly review of the scientific knowledge has been undertaken and translated into language that every person can understand. Her personal anecdotes reveal that hormonal dysfunction can affect us all, and more importantly can now be successfully corrected in very many cases.

This book is essential reading for women of all ages, **and** their male partners.

Doctor Oscar Horky is a specialist obstetrician and gynaecologist.

INTRODUCTION

Hormones are beyond a doubt the most powerful chemicals in your body. They have the power to be physically and emotionally shattering or they can make you feel wonderfully alive. No-one wants to live on a series of extreme highs or lows and we don't have to do that anymore because it's now possible to fine-tune your hormones to avoid this "hormonal seesaw". To feel really well most of the time you need to achieve a balance in your hormones and this book teaches you how. Thousands of women feel trapped and scared and, as victims of their hormones, are desperately searching for ways to escape the prison of hormonal chaos.

We will look at how hormones affect your mental and emotional state, your nerves, sexuality, skin, hair loss, weight, body shape, ageing, the menstrual cycle, headaches and your energy. We will resolve your dilemmas about the oral contraceptive pill and tubal ligation.

This book is not for women only, but contains issues of vital concern for men as well. For too long the "male menopause" has been ignored, denied or embarrassingly hushed up. Men aren't supposed to have such problems and often are told that their midlife crisis is all in the mind even though the reality is that they too can have devastating hormonal imbalances. Thankfully, modern Hormone Replacement Therapy holds the promise of cures for men as much as it does for women.

This handbook gives you the tools to gain control of your hormones which will free you to realise your full potential and enjoy good health. With the right information you need not let your hormones ruin your life.

This book is dedicated to my two grandmothers
Rosina Adelaide McRae and Suzannah Dalton
who were both strong and inspiring women
ahead of their time.

DIAGRAM 1: ENDOCRINE GLANDS AND THEIR HORMONES

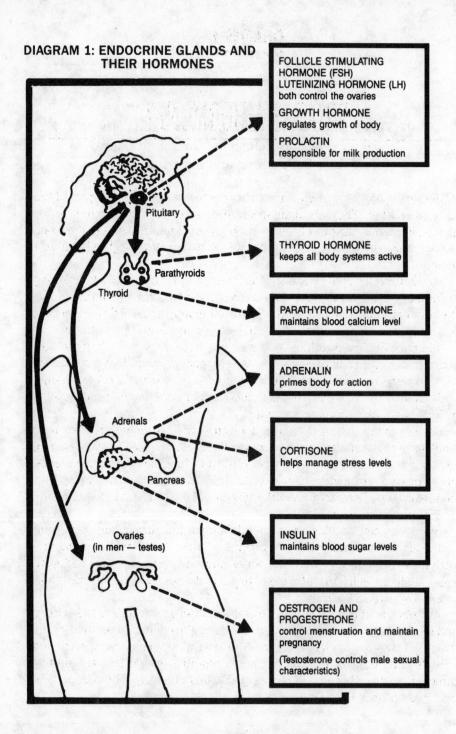

FOLLICLE STIMULATING HORMONE (FSH)
LUTEINIZING HORMONE (LH)
both control the ovaries

GROWTH HORMONE
regulates growth of body

PROLACTIN
responsible for milk production

THYROID HORMONE
keeps all body systems active

PARATHYROID HORMONE
maintains blood calcium level

ADRENALIN
primes body for action

CORTISONE
helps manage stress levels

INSULIN
maintains blood sugar levels

OESTROGEN AND PROGESTERONE
control menstruation and maintain pregnancy

(Testosterone controls male sexual characteristics)

Pituitary

Parathyroids

Thyroid

Adrenals

Pancreas

Ovaries
(in men — testes)

CHAPTER 1

WHAT IS A HORMONE?

Hormones are body chemicals that carry messages from one part of the body to another. They are manufactured in specialised glands (endocrine glands) located in various places in our body and are circulated in the blood to body cells where their presence makes a dramatic impact. (See Diagram 1 opposite).

Some examples of the many glands required to keep our cells functioning in harmony are: the thyroid gland which manufactures thyroid hormone, the adrenal glands which manufacture adrenalin and cortisone and the ovaries which produce the sex hormones oestrogen and progesterone.

Compared to many other body systems, hormones are relatively slow acting in their function of controlling the chemistry of cells. Hormones determine the rate at which our cells burn up food substances and release energy and also determine what metabolic product our cells should produce such as milk, hair, secretions or enzymes.

Hormones are extremely potent molecules and in some cases less than a millionth of a gram is enough to trigger their effects. They are far too small to be seen even under a microscope. After they have completed their tasks, hormones are broken down by the cells themselves or are carried to the liver for breakdown. They are then either excreted or used again to manufacture new hormone molecules.

Hormones can be likened to chemical keys that turn vitally important metabolic locks in our cells. The turning of these locks stimulates activity within the cells of our brain, intestines, muscles, genital organs and skin. Indeed, all our cells are influenced to some degree by these amazing hormonal keys. (See Diagram 2).

Without the hormonal keys the metabolic locks on our cells remain closed and the full potential of our cells is not realised. Imagine a corporation where the employees are unable to communicate with the managing director and are left to do their own thing. Such a corporation would lack any unified direction or growth and the resulting chaos is precisely what happens in our cells without hormones.

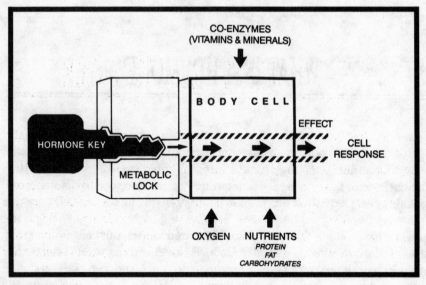

DIAGRAM 2

CHAPTER 2

THE PRE-MENSTRUAL SYNDROME

Katrina had married at the age of 19 against the advice of parents and friends. By the age of 22 she had two beautiful toddlers and a successful husband who doted on his children. Katrina should have been blissfully happy, but she wasn't. For two weeks before her periods, she became morose, irritable and hurtful to her family. She lost interest in sex and felt ugly and unloved. When her menstrual flow began, the dark clouds dissolved and she became her carefree self again but with bitter memories of how she had hurt those she loved. She became the caring mother and wife and resumed her painting and pottery as an expression of her creative spirit. Life was good again up until ovulation began and then, with monotonous regularity, the dark storm clouds gathered around.

Bettina, aged 37 had a vastly different lifestyle to Katrina. She was the typical 20th-century career woman, an executive in a multi-national corporation. She told her friends that she had simply forgotten to have children and marriage was not on her agenda in the context of her sixty-five-hour working week. There were many who envied her, but underneath her cool executive veneer, Bettina was starting to crack. She jumped down the throats of her colleagues, mixed up appointments and became confused for about seven days before each period. She made obvious and serious mistakes and blamed others for not covering up for her inadequacies. The only way Bettina could cope during the week before her period, was by drinking more alcohol and chain-smoking. She was wracked by vascular-tension headaches for three days before her periods and needed frequent doses of painkillers to keep going. As soon as her period began, her headaches vanished and she became once again the cool, calm, collected executive with the seemingly perfect veneer. Deep down Bettina knew that if this monthly imbalance continued she would be burnt out by the age of 45.

Perhaps you can see yourself in these two very different women. As a doctor I see hundreds of such cases in my surgery every year. It is the classic, woeful tale of pre-menstrual syndrome or PMS. Most women will have heard of PMS as it has received extensive coverage in the press and media, but it still remains a misunderstand and poorly treated issue.

15

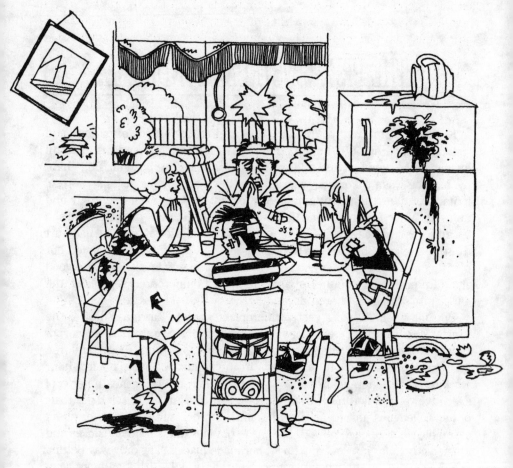

"*. . . and we are especially thankful that Mummy's period is over for another month.*"

PMS is surprisingly common and surprisingly variable. About 50% of women in their reproductive years will notice unpleasant mental and physical changes in themselves sometime in the two weeks before the menstrual bleeding begins.

PMS is the medical term used to describe the collection of different mental and physical problems that may occur during the second half of the menstrual cycle. There are many different problems and symptoms and the important clue is not their nature but the cyclical timing of the symptoms.

If the symptoms are due to PMS, they will begin in the second half of the monthly menstrual cycle, sometime after ovulation and will disappear once the menstrual flow begins. The symptoms will then reappear after ovulation occurs in the next menstrual cycle and so the cyclical repetitive nature of PMS will become apparent. (See Diagram 3). Some women will notice symptoms for the full two weeks preceeding bleeding while others will feel unwell for only several days before bleeding. Some months may be worse than others with a variation in the intensity and type of symptoms.

There are many possible symptoms of PMS and indeed Dr. Katharina Dalton, a world authority on this subject has identified 150 of them. Once again, it is not the type of symptoms but the cyclical relationship of the symptoms before menstrual bleeding that distinguishes PMS from other medical disorders.

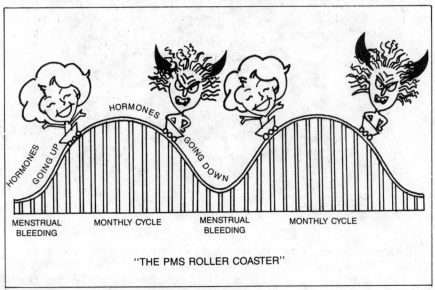

"THE PMS ROLLER COASTER"

DIAGRAM 3: THE PMS ROLLER COASTER

WHAT ARE THE MOST COMMON SYMPTOMS OF THE PMS
Mental and Psychological

Depression, anxiety, irritability, sudden mood changes, aggression, hostility, alcoholic bouts, drug abuse, panic attacks, insomnia, fatigue, sleepiness, confusion, low self-esteem, paranoia, reduced concentration, exhaustion, changes in libido. Some of the more curious symptoms include creative urges or feeling 'spaced out'.

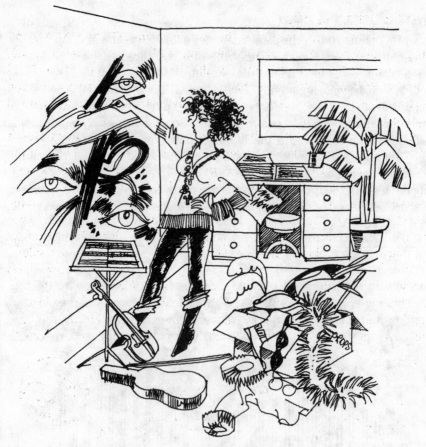

Some of the more curious symptoms of the PMS include creative urges . . .

Physical

Headaches, breast swelling and tenderness, fluid retention, bloating, low blood sugar, food cravings, sugar binges, dramatic changes in weight, clumsiness, poor co-ordination, fainting, acne, general aches and pains, backaches, muscle tension and spasm, constipation and pelvic pain.

Another curious phenomenon is that of "pre-menstrual magnification". This means that medical problems such as allergies, mouth ulcers, genital herpes, candida, asthma, epilepsy, schizophrenia, arthritis, etc., may become worse during the two pre-menstrual weeks. During this time there seems to be a reduction in the general resistance and efficiency of several body systems. If you have an achilles heel, it is most likely to affect you in this pre-menstrual zone.

WHAT CAUSES THE PMS?

I well remember one evening in the country town of Grafton, NSW, relating the Hippocrates theory on the causation of PMS to an entirely male audience who had come to listen to my after-dinner talk about "How To Be A Perfect Husband". My mother had got me into this rather sticky situation as she had delighted in "setting me up" when the Lions Club had requested my presence.

As I related that Hippocrates had blamed a wandering uterus that travelled up to the brain and disturbed the emotions, a little man at the back of the audience became wide-eyed and intrigued. I further related that Hippocrates' treatment for PMS was to entice the wayward uterus back into its rightful position in the pelvis by burning aromatic incense at the vaginal opening. At this juncture the same man's jaw fell open and he looked relieved. After my light-hearted dissertation, he came to me and whispered in my ear saying that he had problems at home and did I have any incense for sale!

After Hippocrates, it took until 1931 for doctors to realise that hormones had something to do with PMS and a certain Dr. Franks preached the theory that too much oestrogen caused PMS. His treatment was more drastic than that of Hippocrates as he recommended large doses of laxatives to flush the demon hormones out of the body. Dr. Franks claimed great success with

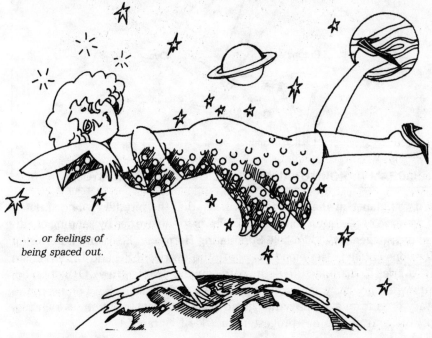

. . . or feelings of being spaced out.

this treatment which is little wonder as the violence of the resulting diar-rhoea was enough to drown out all the other woes of the PMS victim.

Some women even had their ovaries subjected to radiation and consequent destruction in a desperate attempt to end their PMS.

There is no doubt that the cyclical fluctuations in the levels of the sex hormones oestrogen and progesterone manufactured by the sex glands (ovaries) play a large role in causing PMS. This is supported by the observation that PMS begins only after puberty, recurs on a monthly basis and disappears during pregnancy and after the menopause.

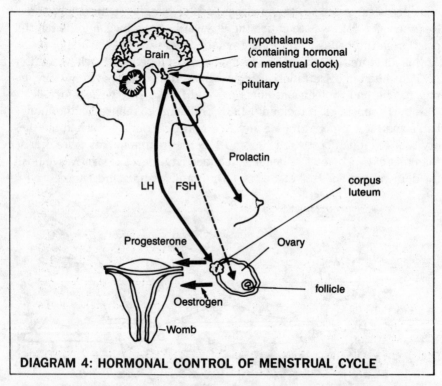

DIAGRAM 4: HORMONAL CONTROL OF MENSTRUAL CYCLE

If you glance at Diagram 4 you will see that the pituitary gland situated at the base of the brain controls and speaks to the ovaries by sending chemical messengers called Follicle Stimulating Hormone (FSH) and Luteinising Hormone (LH) via the blood stream to the ovaries. FSH and LH stimulate the ovaries to manufacture both oestrogen and progesterone. Ovulation occurs when an ovary releases a mature egg and the cells left behind in the ovary then form a small yellow gland called the corpus luteum which sets to work and pumps out progesterone. (See Diagram 5).

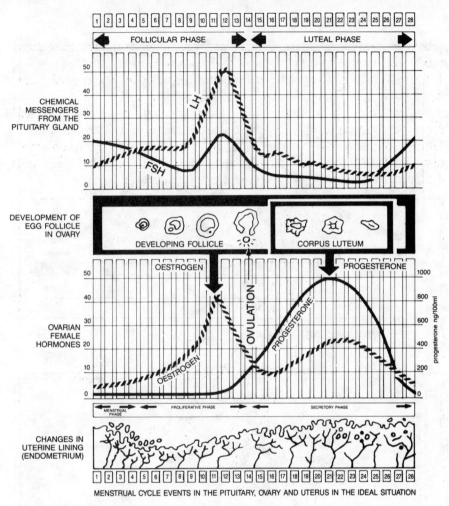

CHEMICAL MESSENGERS FROM THE PITUITARY GLAND

DEVELOPMENT OF EGG FOLLICLE IN OVARY

DEVELOPING FOLLICLE / CORPUS LUTEUM

OVARIAN FEMALE HORMONES

OESTROGEN / PROGESTERONE / OVULATION

CHANGES IN UTERINE LINING (ENDOMETRIUM)

MENSTRUAL PHASE / PROLIFERATIVE PHASE / SECRETORY PHASE

MENSTRUAL CYCLE EVENTS IN THE PITUITARY, OVARY AND UTERUS IN THE IDEAL SITUATION

FSH = Follicle Stimulating Hormone
LH = Luteinising Hormone

DIAGRAM 5: NORMAL MENSTRUAL CYCLE EVENTS IN THE PITUITARY, OVARY AND UTERUS

It is after ovulation in PMS sufferers that the fireworks begin. (See Diagram 6). In a woman without PMS, the levels of oestrogen and progesterone remain in sufficient and balanced amounts between ovulation and menstrual bleeding. In a woman with PMS, the levels of oestrogen and progesterone are out of balance with insufficient oestrogen and/or progesterone between ovulation and bleeding. (See Diagram 6).

Some researchers believe that it is the ratio of oestrogen to progesterone that is more important than the absolute amounts of these hormones. They

DON'T LET YOUR HORMONES RUIN YOUR LIFE

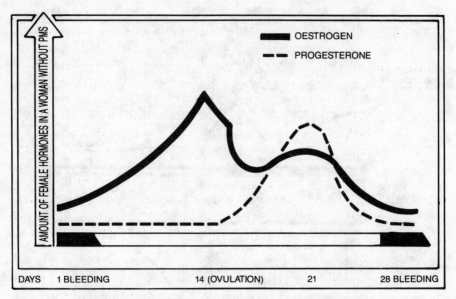

NORMAL MENSTRUAL CYCLE — WITHOUT PMS

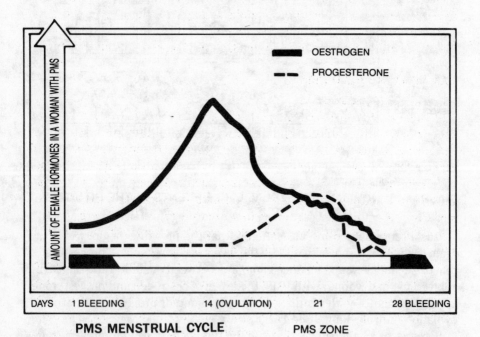

PMS MENSTRUAL CYCLE   PMS ZONE

DIAGRAM 6

have found that women who have too much oestrogen compared to progesterone have anxiety, while women with too little oestrogen compared to progesterone complain of depression during the premenstrual phase.

Indeed, there are many subtle variations in the levels of sex hormones produced from the ovaries and a whole range of imbalances in all three ovarian sex hormones, oestrogen, progesterone and testosterone are probably involved. This accounts for the variation in PMS symptoms between different women and between different cycles in the same woman.

The study of female sex hormones is called gynaecological endocrinology and it is a relatively new medical specialty with still much to explore and learn. We stand at the frontier of an explosion in the understanding and scientific discovery of how imbalances in sex hormones influence our mind and bodies. PMS is truly a Pandora's box and we have now dared to lift the lid so that one by one the hormonal demons will be tamed and controlled.

DOES NUTRITION PLAY A ROLE IN PMS?

Nutritional imbalances and deficiencies can greatly worsen PMS. I have observed that many women obtain complete relief from PMS after improving their diet and/or taking nutritional supplements. You may, as I did originally, find it surprising that such simple and safe nutritional strategies can completely overcome the sometimes dramatic and severe symptoms of hormonal imbalance and yet it is a demonstrated fact that I have seen countless times.

CAN VITAMINS HELP PMS?

Vitamin B6 (Pyridoxine)

A number of studies have found that vitamin B6 in a daily dosage of 25mg to 100mg can give satisfactory relief of many PMS symptoms such as premenstrual headaches, fluid retention, irritability and depression in around 60% to 80% of women. (References 7, 8, 9). Vitamin B6 helps to regulate the brain's biochemistry and is necessary for the conversion of tryptophan to the brain hormone serotonin. Serotonin is a natural regulator of mood, sex drive, sleep and appetite. In my experience, vitamin B6 is more effective if it is taken along with other B complex vitamins such as vitamin B1 (thiamine) 50mg and vitamin B3 (niacinamide) 100mg daily.

I had the pleasure of discussing women's health with the remarkable doctor, Lady Cilento, shortly before her death and she told me that she had had great success in alleviating PMS in thousands of women with one injection every four weeks of vitamin B12 (cyanocobalamin). This certainly has merit in women with poor diets, heavy menstrual bleeding or in those who are strict vegetarians or suffer with digestive complaints.

One of the antioxidants, **vitamin E** can also be most helpful because it is involved in the production of various hormones from the adrenal and pituitary glands as well as the vitally important male hormones. Vitamin E is a superb antioxidant protecting the fatty membranes of our cells thereby improving ovarian function and reducing inflammation. Several studies have found it successful in relieving premenstrual breast pain and lumpiness. (References 10 & 11).

CAN NUTRITIONAL MINERALS HELP PMS?

Zinc

Zinc plays a vital role in human metabolism and has been found to be commonly deficient in the diets of western women in the reproductive age group. Zinc is necessary for proper function of the ovaries, a healthy immune system and skeleton and it promotes strong and healthy skin and hair. It could be considered a mineral to enhance physical beauty and many PMS sufferers should take a regular supplement of zinc. (See Table 1).

Magnesium

This mineral is often deficient in women who consume a diet that is high in refined carbohydrate and sugar. Such a diet will deplete the body of the minerals chromium, manganese, zinc and magnesium and the B complex vitamins. Women with PMS have been found to have lower levels of magnesium in their red blood cells, compared to PMS-free women. (Reference 12). Women with a magnesium deficiency often crave sugar and in particular, chocolate which is a source of dietary magnesium, albeit a poor one. I have found that many chocoholics can easily resist chocolate binges after commencing a magnesium supplement.

Other Important Minerals that may help PMS are chromium, manganese and iron. These are helpful for women with unstable blood sugar levels which cause mood changes, light headedness and sugar cravings, particularly if a meal is missed. (See Table 1). An iron supplement should be taken by all women with heavy menstrual bleeding especially if they are vegetarian. Some women are unable to tolerate inorganic iron which may cause nausea, constipation, cramps and blackening of the bowel action because of poor absorption. In such cases, I suggest an organic iron supplement such as "Hemofactor" available from the pharmacy. All iron supplements are best taken on an empty stomach with vitamin C or citrus fruit to aid absorption.

For those women particularly interested in mineral deficiencies and imbalances, a mineral analysis of your hair can be done to determine the mineral balance of your body. (See Reference 13).

TABLE 1: PMS NATUROPATHIC TREATMENT

REMEDY	ACTION	BENEFIT	DOSAGE (DAILY)
Vitamins			
B1, B3, B6, B12	Essential for metabolism of body and nervous system.	Reduce mood disorders. Increase energy and mental efficiency.	B$_1$ 50mg, B$_3$ 100mg, B$_6$ 25mg, B$_{12}$ 25mcg
A and E	Anti-oxidants, aid ovarian function.	Reduce breast pain. Improve skin, circulation and exercise performance.	Vit E 50iu Vit A 2000iu
Minerals			
Zinc, magnesium, manganese, chromium, iron.	Stabilise blood sugar level, essential for cellular metabolism and immune function.	Reduce craving for sugar and junk foods, improves hair and nails, reduces fatigue. Iron reduces anaemia.	Zinc 30 to 50mg. Magnesium 50mg (varies, may be more) Manganese 5mg Chromium 0.5mg Iron 100 to 200mg
Herbs			
Agnus castus (chaste tree) Helonias (false unicorn root)	Aids ovarian function. Aids ovarian function.	Reduces PMS Reduces PMS, esp. good after stopping OCP.	Agnus Castus and Helonias: dried fruit ½-1gm by infusion as herbal tea. Tincture 1:5 in 45% alcohol, 1-5ml daily
Turnera Diffusa (Damiana)	Tonic for nervous system.	Reduces depression, improves libido.	Damiana : dried leaves 2-4gm by infusion as tea. Tincture 1:5 in 40% alcohol, 1-2ml daily
Essential Fatty Acids (EFAs)			
Evening Primrose Oil (Omega 6)	Balance prostaglandins, reduce inflammation	Improve skin, hair and nails. Reduces breast pains, headaches and other musculoskeletal aches and pains.	Evening Primrose Oil, 1000 to 3000 mg daily
Borage Oil (Omega 6)	Improve function of ovaries and immune system	May help those with pelvic inflammation due to endometriosis or pelvic inflammatory disease.	Borage Oil capsules 600-1000 mg daily
Fish Oil (Omega 3)	Balance prostaglandins, reduce inflammation	Often reduces period pains.	Fish Oil 1000mg daily

Recommended Brands:

Femme Phase contains herbal oestrogens combined with calcium, magnesium, B complex vitamins and foods containing phytoestrogens. It can be stirred into fresh juices. Organic mineral complex. Naudicelle evening primrose oil. AMCAL PMT formula.

Essential Fatty Acids

The dietary essential fatty acids are the building blocks for a very powerful group of hormone-like chemicals in our body called "prostaglandins". Prostaglandins regulate many vital body functions such as hormone production, circulation, immune function and inflammation, just to name a few! It is helpful for you to know that there are three different families of prostaglandins and the prostaglandin 2 family promotes inflammation and pain, whereas the prostaglandin 1 and prostaglandin 3 families reduce inflammation and pain. (At least, it's 2 to 1 in favour of the good guys). See Table 2 to see what foods provide you with certain essential fatty acids which in turn are used to form prostaglandins.

Doctors frequently prescribe the powerful anti-prostaglandin drugs which suppress production of all three families of prostaglandins (good and bad alike) and that is why there are sometimes side effects from these drugs. These drugs are called anti-inflammatory drugs (examples are indocid, naprogesic, ponstan) and can be very effective in stopping the pain and inflammation of headaches, arthritis and period pains.

I have found that in many cases of PMS, headaches, or period pains, it is possible to rebalance the three prostaglandin families simply by changing the diet and taking supplements of essential fatty acids. This reduces pain and inflammation in a natural way.

To reduce the amounts of the undesirable prostaglandin 2 family, you should reduce saturated fats and fried foods.

To increase the amounts of the desirable prostaglandin 1 and prostaglandin 3 families, you should consume a diet that is high in seeds, vegetables, fish and polyunsaturated oils. (See Table 2).

Another efficient way to balance the prostaglandin families is to take supplements of essential fatty acids. The best known one is evening primrose oil (EPO) which contains the essential fatty acids linoleic acid and gamma linolenic acid (GLA). GLA can be hard to come by in a normal western diet (See Table 2), the highest source being found in breast milk, which partly explains why breast-fed babies are generally healthier than bottle-fed babies. EPO will increase the prostaglandin 1 family and can be remarkably effective in reducing pre-menstrual headaches, arthritis, breast tenderness, period pains and other symptoms of PMS. EPO is helpful for ovarian function and helps to return regularity to the menstrual cycle and reduces ovarian cysts.

My sister, Madeleine, an actress, finds it superb for her hair and skin and says that she is happy to go without several of life's little luxuries provided she can have her capsules of EPO. Initial doses of EPO required may be quite high ranging from six to nine capsules daily, however, after six to eight weeks

TABLE 2

Foods ►	Essential Fatty Acids ►	Prostaglandin Family ►	Effect In Body
Sesame, Sunflower seeds and oil, cold-pressed vegetable oils (polyunsaturated), blackcurrant seeds and their oil, evening primrose oil, borage oil	Linoleic acid, ► Gamma linolenic acid	Prostaglandin 1 (desirable)	Reduces pain and inflammation
Saturated animal fats in animal meats, (especially red meat) full-cream dairy products, preserved meats, fried foods, processed and take away meals	Arachidonic ► acid	Prostaglandin 2 (undesirable)	Increases pain and inflammation, can result in sticky platelets and poor circulation
Linseed oil, blackcurrant seeds and their oil, cod liver oil, mackerel and fresh fish (from cold deep oceans) sardines, tuna, salmon, (must not be fried)	Alpha linolenic ► acid, eicosapentaenoic acid (EPA)	Prostaglandin 3 (desirable)	Reduces pain and inflammation

a maintenance dose of two to four capsules daily usually keeps PMS under control.

Supplements of fish oil, linseed oil and blackcurrant seed oil will increase the production of the desirable prostaglandin 3 family which is helpful in reducing many PMS type symptoms. (See Table 2). For those who don't like to swallow too many capsules a potent source of the precious essential fatty acid GLA is available in the form of "Super Naudicelle" capsules which contain EPO, borage oil and fish oil. If you have trouble absorbing or tolerating capsules of essential fatty acids, EPO is available in a non-oily and highly absorbed liquid form — "EPO Micelle".

THE ANTI-PMS DIET — GOLDEN RULES

There are a few golden rules to follow and if you observe them six days a week, you will be able to enjoy the occasional indiscretion with impunity and a clear conscience.

GOLDEN RULES	GOOD EFFECTS
Avoid refined carbohydrates, soft drinks and refined sugars. Get your sugar from fresh fruits.	Aids weight control, stabilises blood sugar levels.
Reduce saturated fats e.g., fatty meats, preserved meats or fried foods, processed and takeaway meals.	Aids weight control, reduces hormonal imbalances, reduces cancer, reduces inflammation and pain.
Reduce salt, caffeine, chocolate and alcohol.	Reduces fluid retention, headaches and breast pain.
Increase foods high in magnesium and iron e.g., whole grains, green leafy vegetables, spinach, cereals, legumes, liver.	Reduces headaches and increases energy levels.
Eat more frequent meals containing first class protein, e.g., eggs, low fat dairy products, fish, seafoods, lean meat. An excellent source of first class protein and fibre is obtained by combining three of the following at one meal — grains, nuts, seeds, legumes.	Stabilises blood sugar level, prevents sugar and junk food binges, increases energy levels.

CAN LIFESTYLE CHANGES HELP PMS?

A reasonably healthy lifestyle is a must if you are serious about beating PMS. Let's check out the benefits of some good habits.

LIFESTYLE	BENEFITS
A regular exercise programme, with some aerobic exercise, some muscle building and relaxing exercise.	Reduces muscle spasm and tension, increases brain endorphins which are natural euphorics, improves blood supply to hormonal glands.
Quit smoking.	Nicotine constricts blood vessels and reduces the blood supply to ovaries. Giving up smoking will increase the hormone output, (especially oestrogen) from your ovaries.
Increase water intake to 2 to 4 litres daily.	Aids weight control and reduces headaches, skin problems and breast pain. Increases energy levels.
Reduce alcohol intake during the two pre-menstrual weeks.	Avoids embarrassing moments. There is a reduced tolerance to alcohol pre-menstrually with higher blood alcohol levels being attained quickly.

The tools of a healthy diet, lifestyle and nutritional supplements will provide relief for the vast majority of women with mild to moderate PMS. Patience and persistence are vital as with most types of nutritional medicine, there is a time lapse of six to eight weeks before major improvements are attained.

WHAT RISK FACTORS INCREASE YOUR CHANCES OF PMS?

1. Family History

You won't thank your ancestors for this familial trait, but there is no doubt that if your mother, sisters or maternal or paternal grandmother or great grandmothers had PMS, then you are also more prone to suffer with PMS.

2. Hormonal Triggers

Many women first notice PMS after stopping the oral contraceptive pill, after pregnancy, postnatal depression or miscarriage, after hysterectomy with conservation of the ovaries or after tubal ligation (sterilization).

Some women get PMS type symptoms while taking the oral contraceptive pill (OCP) presumably because the synthetic hormones in the OCP reduce the production of natural oestrogen and progesterone from the ovaries. If this is severe, a progesterone only OCP (mini-pill) may be better tolerated.

3. Stress

PMS may appear after severe or prolonged stress, such as relationship difficulties, financial problems or unwanted pregnancies.

4. Increasing Age

Typically PMS worsens during the 30s, peaking in the mid to late 30s. During the 40s, PMS becomes intertwined with the hormonal deficiencies characteristic of the pre-menopausal years when more severe deficiencies and/or imbalances of oestrogen and progesterone can occur.

5. Being A 20th Century Woman

Today's woman has, on average, two children and spends the rest of her life having regular menstrual cycles with approximately 350 to 400 menstrual periods in her reproductive life span. Therefore, if she is susceptible, she could have 350 to 400 episodes of PMS in her lifetime. Before contraception was available, a woman had around ten pregnancies, each followed by one to two years of breast-feeding. Our great grandmothers usually only menstruated for two to five years out of their whole life span. Thus, as far as mother nature is concerned, it would seem that women are not meant to have periods and PMS, and that they are indeed designed to have more pregnancies.

IS THERE A TEST FOR PMS?

The most accurate way to determine if you have PMS is to keep a menstrual calendar on which you chart the timing of your symptoms and menstrual bleeding. It is not the type of symptoms that is important, but rather the fact that your symptoms recur every month, some time after ovulation and are relieved when menstrual bleeding is well under way. The chart of Maggie (opposite) illustrates a classic tale of PMS and there is a table for you to photocopy and use to chart your own symptoms on Page 32. Keep your chart

MAGGIE'S CHART

	January	February	March	April
1		H B D	M	
2	B	M P	M	
3	B	M P	M	
4	B	M		
5	H B D	M		
6	H B D	M		
7	H B D			
8	M P			
9	M P			
10	M			
11	M			
12	M			D
13				B D
14				B D
15				B D
16				B D
17				H B D
18				M P
19			D	M
20			B D	M
21			B D	M
22		D	H B D	M
23		B D	H B D	
24		H B D	M P	
25		H B D	M P	
26		H B D	M	
27	B	M P	M	
28	B	M	M	
29	B D			
30	H B D			
31	H B D			

CODE: M = menstrual bleeding   D = depression   H = headache
B = breast pain   P = period pain

Maggie has a 5 day bleeding cycle approximately every 25 days.

YOUR MENSTRUAL CALENDAR

	Jan	Feb	Mar	Apr	May	Jun	Jul	Aug	Sep	Oct	Nov	Dec
1												
2												
3												
4												
5												
6												
7												
8												
9												
10												
11												
12												
13												
14												
15												
16												
17												
18												
19												
20												
21												
22												
23												
24												
25												
26												
27												
28												
29												
30												
31												

On this chart mark the days of menstrual bleeding with an 'M' and the days of your MOST IMPORTANT SYMPTOMS with an appropriate symbol, eg:
H = headache   B = bloatedness/water retention   BT = breast tenderness
D = depression   I = irritability   P = period pains
or invent symbols for your priority symptoms. Even if you are not menstruating, eg. have had a hysterectomy, it will help your doctor if you chart the dates of your symptoms.

for three months and then take it along to your doctor to enable an accurate diagnosis of your hormonal balance or imbalance, as the case may be.

Generally speaking, expensive blood tests to measure hormone levels are not necessary but if your doctor is unsure of the diagnosis or if a serious hormonal imbalance is suspected then blood tests are necessary. It is best to measure blood hormone levels when you feel at your best and again at your worst, as determined by your menstrual calendar. This will pinpoint exactly what type of hormonal imbalance you could have.

THE STORY OF PAULA

In its most severe manifestation the pre-menstrual syndrome is a disorder that can ruin your life. This was brought home to me one day by a 42-year-old librarian called Paula who came to see me as her last hope. Paula had first noticed severe mood changes before menstruation, shortly after an early puberty at the age of 10. By the age of 18, her pre-menstrual depression was so severe that she attempted suicide with an overdose of her mother's sedatives. She was diagnosed as manic-depressive and prescribed the drug Lithium. This reduced her mood swings, but she still felt unwell with headaches, bloating, sore breasts and extreme fatigue for ten days before her menstrual bleeding. Paula was gradually taken off Lithium so that she could become pregnant and by the third month of her pregnancy, she felt wonderful. She said "For the first time in my life, I feel in control, peaceful and free of headaches and I love the feeling of those huge amounts of hormones filling up my body". Paula had a natural birth and things were going well until six weeks after childbirth, severe postnatal depression began. Paula again attempted suicide and was again prescribed Lithium. Twelve months later at the age of 31, Paula, terrified of another episode of postnatal depression, begged for sterilization by having her tubes tied (tubal ligation). After consulting six gynaecologists, the tubal ligation was unfortunately performed and, not surprisingly, she then began to experience severe PMS. For twelve days before every period she felt dead and found herself in a deep pit of depression and anger. Her head ached, her abdomen swelled and she became aggressive with her husband and child. Paula felt trapped knowing that every month after ovulation she would feel as if a switch inside her brain turned on producing volcanic changes in her personality and body. Once her menstrual bleeding started, the switch would be turned off and the depression, aggression and headaches would miraculously vanish. After menstruation she felt in control, but was haunted by feelings of remorse and guilt for the disruption she had caused. Her husband could recognise the night and day effect caused by this hormonal switch and he could see that she needed help. Paula visited eight different gynaecologists and tried diuretics, sedatives, anti-depressants, the oral contraceptive pill, synthetic progesterone, psychotherapy and chiropractic treatment. In a desperate attempt to save her marriage she asked for a hysterectomy and reluctantly, feeling that she had tried all possible therapies, her last doctor removed her uterus.

Paula felt better for three months after her hysterectomy until during the fourth month she noticed that her depression and anger returned for two weeks. For the next six months she found that for two weeks out of every four she was again in the grip of severe mood changes. She returned to the doctor begging to have her ovaries removed. Thankfully, this time the doctor refused and referred her to a psychiatrist.

Paula had classic PMS in a severe degree and was in urgent need of natural hormone therapy. Her hysterectomy had relieved her headaches and fatigue but had done nothing to quell the cyclical surges and falls of sex hormones from her ovaries. She felt great when her ovaries were pumping out oestrogen and progesterone and terrible when they stopped. Paula's case supports the research finding that when the uterus is removed and the ovaries left in place, the symptoms and hormonal changes of PMS may persist, although often to a lesser degree. (Reference 2).

I suggested to Paula that her brain would function properly if we maintained a stable and adequate level of the natural oestrogen, oestradiol, in her blood every day. She willingly accepted an initial course of natural oestrogen injections followed up with an implant of natural oestrogen. Three months later Paula felt civilised and happy again and remarked that the constant hormone levels in her blood provided by her oestrogen implant made her feel the way she felt during pregnancy. Paula could now cope, and every day was cool. She felt as if a prison door had been unlocked and she would no longer be trapped in a vicious hormone cycle. Such can be the drama of severe PMS.

Women are "hormonal creatures", riding upon the waves of hormonal surges and indeed this is largely responsible for the alluring mystery that womanhood presents to males. However, for a significant percentage of women, the price of this hormonal uniqueness is too much to pay. **Thankfully, we no longer have to be victims of wild hormonal imbalances as modern day hormonal therapy can re-programme our hormonal cycle. One could say the self-programmable bionic woman has arrived!**

HORMONAL TREATMENTS FOR PMS

In severe cases of PMS that do not respond to diet and nutritional supplements, corrective hormonal therapy can be life-saving. If PMS is so severe that it is associated with uncontrollable mood changes, reduced ability to function, thoughts of suicide, marital disruption, child abuse or dangerous behaviour, then hormonal therapy is usually required to restore equanimity. Many of these women have been offered sedatives, anti-depressants and counselling and come along to the doctor desperately hoping that hormonal help will be at hand. Thankfully, it is and is often dramatically effective.

Progesterone

The use of natural progesterone has been popularised and advocated by Dr. Katharina Dalton, who is somewhat of a "PMS guru" and she has shown it to be effective in relieving most types of PMS. (References 3, 4, 5). Progesterone appears useful in relieving pre-menstrual depression, anxiety, mood changes, fatigue and low blood sugar levels and may reduce menstrual bleeding.

It is important to realise that Dr. Dalton only recommends the use of natural progesterone with a chemical structure identical to the progesterone produced by the ovaries. Natural progesterone is made from soya beans and sweet potatoes (yams).

Unfortunately, doctors often prescribe strong synthetic progesterones called "progestogens" for PMS sufferers, mistakenly believing that they will have the same effect as natural progesterone. This is not true and many of these synthetic progestogens are derived from male (testosterone-like) synthetic hormones and so may cause side effects such as increased appetite, weight gain, fluid retention, acne, greasy skin and increased cholesterol. These synthetic progestogen hormones fit into the natural progesterone receptors found throughout the body and brain but cannot turn or switch on these receptors. Only natural progesterone can turn on the progesterone receptors just as a key turns and releases a lock. So you can understand that synthetic progestogens will not have the same beneficial effect as natural progesterone and indeed many PMS sufferers feel more depressed and tired when they take them.

The progesterone story is very complicated and so I have designed an easy reference table on Pages 36-37 to help you and your doctor understand how to use progesterone for PMS. Unfortunately, natural progesterone is not very effective if taken by mouth (orally) as it is destroyed by the liver enzymes after absorption. Therefore, it needs to be administered by either vaginal pessary, rectal suppository, deep oily intramuscular injection into the buttocks or by natural progesterone implants. By giving natural progesterone in these ways we are bypassing the liver so that the progesterone can be absorbed directly into the circulation and carried to the progesterone receptors on your cells.

TABLE 3: PMS HORMONE TREATMENT CHART

HORMONE	TYPE	DOSAGE	BENEFIT	DRAWBACKS	POSSIBLE SIDE EFFECTS
Progesterone pessaries or suppositories 200mg	Natural	From 1 to 4 daily inserted vaginally or rectally after emptying bladder and bowels. Insert 1 at a time only.	May relieve physical and mental symptoms of PMS.	Wear a pad to avoid leakage. Expensive. For info phone 02 387 3205 or fax 02 389 3821 or contact infertility clinics.	Occasional vaginal/rectal irritation and breakthrough bleeding, delayed onset of menstrual bleeding.
Progesterone injections "Proluton" 25mg	Natural	Intramuscular injection in the buttock 50 to 100mg daily.	More powerful effect than pessaries/suppositories in relieving PMS. Proluton is identical to natural progesterone.	Expensive. Proluton only available in 25mg, may need 100mg Progesterone injection. More available in UK, USA. See Page 144. Oily injections can cause slight discomfort.	Menstrual irregularity breakthrough bleeding, allergic rash, scar tissue or abscess in buttock in long term users is possible.
"Proluton Depot" 250mg	Neutral	250mg as one injection at the time of ovulation i.e. mid cycle.	Proluton Depot is slightly modified but is still free of masculine side-effects and does not reduce production of natural progesterone from ovaries.		
Progesterone implants 200mg	Natural	2 to 5, implants inserted into fat of the buttocks.	Can be excellent if progesterone pessaries or injections gave complete relief. Not messy or uncomfortable.	Expensive. Difficult to obtain.	Menstrual irregularity, infrequent periods or breakthrough bleeding.
Progesterone Lozenges	Natural	100mg, one to three times daily orally.	Can relieve PMS.	Expensive. Contact 02 9387 3205	Breakthrough bleeding.
Progestogens e.g. norethisterone, norgesterol, medroxyprogesterone acetate	Synthetic	Varies depending upon brand of tablet.	Reduces heavy menstrual bleeding and period pains. May reduce breast tenderness.	Do not help emotional or mental problems of PMS.	Some brands may cause weight gain, greasy skin, mood changes, fluid retention. Increased cholesterol.

TABLE 3: PMS HORMONE TREATMENT CHART

Name	Type	Dosage	Benefits	Comments	Side effects
"In-Between Progesterones" Dydrogesterone (Duphaston)	Neutral 'clean' progestogen'	10 to 20mg daily in tablet form from day 12-28 of menstrual cycle.	Several studies in UK and Europe have found it effective in relieving mental and physical symptoms of PMS. Duphaston has a very close chemical structure to natural progesterone and is well absorbed.	Expensive unless you have endometriosis, may not be as good as natural progesterone in relieving mood disorders of PMS.	Very few side effects, that's why its called 'clean' unlike synthetic progestogens. May cause some breakthrough bleeding.
Progesterone patches	Natural or synthetic	Varies	The natural progesterone patch should be the best form of treatment for PMS when it becomes available.	Natural progesterone patches. Unavailable as yet – urgently needed. Synthetic progesterone patches available called Estracombi.	Probably none. Perhaps occasional breakthrough bleeding.
Oral contraceptive pill (OCP)	Synthetic oestrogen and progestogen or progestogen only pill.	As recommended on packet.	Can help some PMS sufferers, reduces menstrual bleeding and pain, regulates menstrual cycle, provides contraception.	Generally does not help mental or emotional problems of PMS, and may worsen these.	May cause headaches, fluid retention and loss of libido, weight gain.
Bromocriptine (Parlodel)	Synthetic hormone which blocks Prolactin secretion from pituitary gland.	1.25-7.5mg daily as tablets.	Relieves severe breast tenderness and pain. No benefit in other PMS symptoms.	Does not help mental symptoms of PMS.	Nausea, headaches, dizziness, fainting.
Oestrogen	Natural, given as tablets, injections, implants or patches.	Varies – determined by your doctor and your age.	May be needed in older women. Improves mood disorders, fatigue, poor libido, rheumatic aches and pains.	May increase menstrual bleeding.	Breast tenderness, fluid retention. Oestrogen tablets may worsen migraine.

FOOTNOTE: Depot = long acting injection lasting for 10 to 14 days.
FOR PRODUCT AVAILABILITY CHART SEE PAGE 144 AND 145.

Neutral progesterone is in between natural and synthetic and is less likely to cause side-effects.
It is imperative that women taking drugs or hormones to treat PMS have adequate means of contraception.

As you can see from Table 3, the use of progesterone is quite complicated and should only be administered under regular medical supervision. In general, progesterone is very safe with side effects such as breakthrough bleeding being of nuisance value only. Pure natural progesterone does not cause birth defects or harm to the foetus if you become pregnant, but unless you are under a specialist for infertility, it is best to avoid all hormones (natural or synthetic) while trying to conceive. Generally, progesterone is started five days before the expected onset of PMS symptoms and continued daily up to the time of expected menstrual bleeding and should prevent most PMS symptoms. Each PMS sufferer is an individual and trial and error using different dosages, forms and schedules of progesterone may be required before the symptoms are under control.

Oestrogens

If progesterone therapy by itself is ineffective for severe PMS, then the use of natural oestrogen may break the cycle of vicious PMS. This is particularly so in older women with PMS whose ovaries are less able to pump out sufficient amounts of oestrogen and also in PMS sufferers who have undergone hysterectomy or tubal ligation. The treatment of PMS with natural oestrogen is similar to the use of natural oestrogen for the menopause. For details on this refer to my book titled *Menopause — You Can Give It A Miss!*

PMS may be relieved by natural oestrogen tablets, injections, implants or patches and you and your doctor may need to try different dosages and forms to get PMS under control.

This was so for 43-year-old Donna, who had first noticed severe PMS eight months after having her tubes tied. Donna was a top marketing executive with many employees under her supervision and she needed her wits about her every day of the month. She was disgusted by the onset of new and strange hormonal upheavals that she described to me as the 'PMT dichotomy'. Donna found that around the sixteenth day of every menstrual cycle she felt like two people inside one body — a kind of Dr. Jekyll and Mrs. Hyde. She described how suddenly she would become irrational and ineffective in the office while another part of her stood by appalled at what the PMS self was doing. She felt out of control until her menstrual bleeding started and then the two Donnas became one peaceful, together person.

Donna knew that she needed hormone therapy as her mental and emotional changes were severe, and her doctor prescribed progesterone pessaries. This took only the edge off her depression and she still felt crazy inside. Donna then began to experience hot flushes and sweating attacks during the week before her menstrual flow. At this time a blood test confirmed low levels of oestrogen and we recognised that her mind and body were crying out for oestrogen. We first tried natural oestrogen tablets which helped the hot flushes but not her mental changes. Finally, much to the relief of Donna and her office staff, I inserted an implant of natural oestrogen which within a week produced a total relief of her mood swings and fatigue.

When it comes to treating pre-menstrual mood swings, depression, fatigue and loss of libido, my preference is to use natural oestrogen implants, injections or patches rather than oestrogen tablets. Implants, injections and patches will produce blood levels of the natural oestrogen "oestradiol" sufficient to suppress the cyclical hormonal highs and lows of the ovaries. Oestradiol is very effective in overcoming depression and loss of libido and oestradiol implants are recommended by Dr. John Studd of St. Thomas Hospital, London, to treat PMS. A trial involving the treatment of fifty women with PMS using oestradiol implants over five to six years found that a beneficial and lasting response occurred in all PMS symptoms with 96% of cases of depression being relieved. (Reference 6).

OTHER DRUGS USED TO TREAT PMS

Can Diuretics Help?

In women with severe premenstrual fluid retention and bloating it may be necessary to use diuretic drugs. Some women find that they retain so much fluid that they gain up to five kilograms of weight during the seven days before menstrual bleeding. This is called cyclical oedema and may be extremely uncomfortable with a new wardrobe being required at this time of the month. In such cases a special diuretic drug called a "potassium sparing diuretic" such as **Moduretic** or **Aldactone** is excellent. These drugs remove unwanted fluid without causing a deficiency of the mineral potassium. Aldactone tablets in a dose of 25 to 100mg twice daily from day 14 to 28 of the menstrual cycle can help reduce depression, fluid retention, acne and greasy skin.

Danazol

Danazol is recommended only for extreme PMS when other drugs and therapies have failed. It is a powerful synthetic steroid hormone with male hormone-like properties. Danazol in a dose of 200-400mg daily suppresses the hormone cycle of the ovary, putting an end to ovulation and menstrual bleeding. It can be effective for PMS, but women often stop taking it because of unacceptable masculine side-effects such as acne, facial hair, weight gain, shrinking breasts and deepening of the voice.

Gonadotrophin Releasing Hormone Agonists (GnRH)

These are powerful synthetic hormones that act on the pituitary gland to completely inhibit the ovarian cycle. Their use results in a "medical menopause'' with very low levels of oestrogen and progesterone and absence of menstrual bleeding. They could only be recommended for severe PMS when all other hormonal and drug therapy has failed and then only on a short-term basis. Their long-term use would result in very low levels of oestrogen with increased risk of osteoporosis and cardiovascular disease.

HOW CAN WE HELP OURSELVES?

I believe that the greatest healer is oneself. To heal ourselves we need to be aware of certain helpful facts and guidelines. Firstly, the understanding that female sex hormone imbalances may play a role in depression is helpful. Women are more prone to depression than men, this depression usually starts after puberty, is worse pre-menstrually, after childbirth and during the zone of the menopausal years. Without this understanding, these disturbances often continue with cyclical regularity and no one does anything effective about it even though disorders like PMS are eminently treatable.

Women need to be aware of the biological model of psychological disorders where it is realised that our state of mind is influenced by our hormones, diet, nutritional status, drugs, lifestyle, general health and the environment and not just psychological factors.

If we can see womanhood as an advantage like a special gift, we are less likely to be intimidated by the cyclic nature of our biology, wanting to explore both its strengths and vulnerabilities. This is easier to enjoy when one knows that if the strengths diminish and the vulnerabilities increase, modern-day hormonal and nutritional therapy can restore the balance.

We need to tap into the wealth of healing resources and knowledge found in our inner selves to keep a balance with our accumulation of scientific and academic facts. By having faith in our inner female intuition we can gain confidence in changing ourselves and any misguided situations around us.

As an academic and eternal medical student, I have kept an open mind about new discoveries and this was partly the reason that I became interested in naturopathic medicine. It seemed to click with my inner sense of intuition and, no matter how much it was ridiculed or minimised by the establishment, it continued to make sense and produce good results. Like all doctors I have accumulated considerable medical wisdom by communicating with my patients, who, together with my intuition, have both taught and inspired me for many years.

WHAT ARE THE OBSTACLES?

The attitude of some drug companies, doctors and psychiatrists is not always conducive to the active participation of women in their health dilemmas.

Some doctors may prefer to keep control by fostering dependent relationships with their patients and keep them "in the dark". Other doctors may be reluctant to accept the biological causes of psychological disorders and there is an urgent need for more interspecialty collaborative research to assess the role of hormones, nutritional supplements and drugs in various types of depression. Some psychiatrists, (usually males), still see women through the teachings of Sigmund Freud who believed that women were inherently more neurotic than men with their inability to resolve subconscious conflicts shown in the typical neuroses of depression, anxiety, hysteria or hypochondriasis. This narrow perspective leads to the stereotyping of women, reinforcing their inferiority and dependence upon mind-altering drugs.

In reality, today's women is psychologically, if not hormonally, just as liberated and aware as today's man. She is increasingly reluctant to accept psychotropic drugs (sedatives, tranquillisers and anti-depressants) for fear that they may take the edge off performance and blunt feelings and self expression.

It is interesting that often it is not only psychiatrists, but also some feminists who are cynical towards the idea that hormone fluctuations affect female psychology and behaviour. Such feminists also have a narrow perspective, preferring to say that the higher incidence of depression and suicide attempts in women is entirely due to environmental and psycho-social issues. They may feel it demeaning or trivialising to admit that one's hormones could wreak mental havoc, fearing that this will give women a handicapping vulnerability or a uniquely female "Achilles heel". This nihilistic attitude of denial is no longer appropriate and hormone therapy will enable us to compete and share with our male counterparts in a world where we need to keep our wits about us not for two, but for four weeks every month.

Another obstacle to overcome is the sometimes confused and crossed messages about our hormones that are given to us by the media, lay press and "pseudo experts" who have never had any clinical experience with women. We read negative and patronising articles with no clear strategies or hopes of cure offered. For example, we are told that PMS women should avoid giving dinner parties at that time of the month as if the most serious implication was a collapsed soufflé or lumpy sauce! This is ineffectual advice for the many professional women of today who are surgeons, airline pilots or politicians.

Another common obstacle is our self-image. Many women have very low self-esteem, and are unable to love and admire themselves as unique individuals and find it uncomfortable to be assertive with their doctors. This lack of confidence makes it difficult for them to express their needs, anger, aggression or resentment especially in front of a professional.

To overcome these limitations, the establishment of support groups for women with such problems as PMS, postnatal depression, drug dependence or midlife depression can be invaluable. Support groups provide an environment where women can begin to express themselves, building skills in confidence, creativity and self-assertiveness. For women who feel they have "lost it", support groups can act as a stepping stone back into the real world. (See Page 150 for a list of support groups).

Support groups can really open other avenues and take on many roles such as sending a spokesperson for a radio interview, writing newspaper articles, inviting an expert speaker on women's health to your area, raising money for the local women's refuge, etc. They also provide psychological support for those women unable to afford expensive counselling from a professional.

At the end of the day we need to keep our sense of humour which can be hard when the struggle for mental and physical harmony seems elusive, so the little cartoons in this chapter will help us to laugh at ourselves. Yes, it's true now, as ever, laughter is a great form of medicine!

REFERENCES

1. Abraham G.E. et al, *Hormonal and behavioural changes during the menstrual cycle*, Senologia. 1978; 3:33.

2. Backstrom C.T., et al, *Persistance of symptoms of PMT in hysterectomised women*, Brit.Journ. Obstets & Gynaec, 1981; 88:530.

3. Dalton K. 1964, *The PMS*, Heinemann, London.

4. Dalton K. 1970, Brit. Med. Journ., 2:27.

5. Dalton K. 1966, Proceedings Royal Society of Medicine, 59: 10, 1014.

6. Watson N.R., et al, Gynaec Endocrinol. 4:99-107, 1990.

7. Taylor, et al, Current Med. Research & Opinion 6, 46-51, 1979.

8. Bavernfeind J.C. *Vit B6: nutritional & pharmaceutical usage*, Pg 78-110, Nat. Acad. of Sciences, Washington 1978.

9. Kerr G.D., Current Med. Opinion & Research, Suppl. 4, Pg 29, 1977.

10. Gordon T., et al, Am. Journ. Med. 62: 707, 1977.

11. Abrams, A.A. New England Journ. Med. 272:1080, 1965.

12. Abraham G., et al, *RBC Magnesium in premenopausal women*, International Clinical Nutrition Review, Vol 3., No. 1, 1983.

13. Hair Analysis Laboratory — Thintron Labs. PO Box 630, Gladesville 2111. Phone: (02) 281 9344.

CHAPTER 3

MENSTRUAL IRREGULARITY

The duration of the menstrual cycle is calculated as the number of days between the first day of bleeding to the first day of bleeding of the next menstrual period. Not every woman has a cycle of exactly 28 days and the normal menstrual cycle can vary from 21 to 35 days.

It is not uncommon for the menstrual periods to become irregular and less frequent. If a woman who previously had regular monthly cycles fails to menstruate for over three months, she has what doctors call amenorrhoea, and this is not a normal state in pre-menopausal women.

WHAT ARE THE CAUSES OF INFREQUENT MENSTRUATION?

In the vast majority of cases a hormonal imbalance resulting in failure to ovulate is the cause, but disorders of the uterus and a possible blockage of the cervix or vagina must be checked. Hormonal imbalances disturb the menstrual clock in the hypothalamus and the sensitive communication link between the hypothalamus, pituitary gland and ovaries. (See Page 20.)

CHANGES IN BODY WEIGHT

The menstrual clock can be switched off by rapid or severe changes in body weight with either weight loss or weight gain having this effect.

Fat produces both female and male sex hormones, and so very thin women have low levels of these hormones. In addition, if the menstrual clock has switched off as a protective mechanism against extreme thinness, ovulation will not occur and so the ovaries will produce very little sex hormones. These low levels of sex hormones cause menstrual bleeding to cease. If weight can be gained to achieve a normal body weight relative to body height, the menstrual clock should restart causing a resumption of regular menstrual bleeding.

Overweight women tend to overproduce female and male sex hormones from their fat. They often have polycystic ovaries (See Page 96) which do not ovulate regularly and produce plenty of oestrogen but insufficient progesterone. They also fail to menstruate regularly as their uterus is exposed to constant high levels of oestrogen. Once again, the achievement of a normal body weight relative to body height (See Opposite) will usually bring back regular ovulation and normal levels of the female and male sex hormones.

WEIGHT FOR HEIGHT (Use this chart to plot weight and progress)

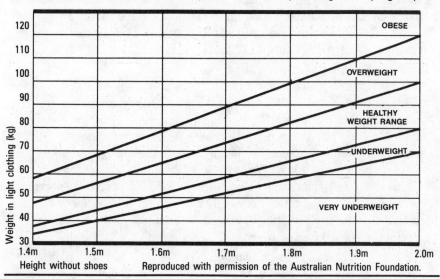

DIAGRAM 19

EXERCISE

Excessive exercise can switch off the menstrual clock resulting in amenorrhoea. Such sportive women may be muscular, but usually have low amounts of fat and thus low levels of sex hormones. If the amenorrhoea persists they will be at a higher risk of osteoporosis despite their vigorous physical workouts.

STRESS

Stress and emotional trauma can act on the hypothalamus to switch off the menstrual clock and in such cases menstruation may not resume until a woman is feeling happy and relaxed. Some women lose their menstrual periods after a traumatic relationship or divorce and find that their periods return when they fall in love again.

IMBALANCE OF THE PITUITARY GLAND

Excessive amounts of the lactation hormone Prolactin, switch off the menstrual clock and the ovaries which is why it is normal for breastfeeding mothers to miss their periods for six months or more.

If a non-lactating woman has excessive Prolactin production from the pituitary gland she may stop menstruating which is not a normal situation. In such cases the excessive Prolactin may result from medications such as anti-depressants or a small tumour in the pituitary gland that overproduces Prolactin. The drug bromocriptine (Parlodel) can correct this situation restoring regular menstruation and fertility.

PREMATURE MENOPAUSE

Some women stop menstruating in their 20s and 30s because of a premature failure of the ovaries. This is called a premature menopause and can be diagnosed with blood tests. These women have used up all the eggs from their ovaries and need to receive Hormone Replacement Therapy (HRT).

In some women menstrual bleeding may not cease altogether, but rather become extremely light with perhaps no more than spotting for a day or so. This is called "hypomenorrhoea". Common causes of hypomenorrhoea are advancing age, weight loss, heavy athletic training or imbalances in other hormonal glands, such as the thyroid or adrenal glands.

TREATMENT OF AMENORRHOEA

If a woman with absent menstruation does not want to become pregnant the best treatment is the Oral Contraceptive Pill (OCP). This will restore regular menstruation and protect the bones from osteoporosis in the underweight woman with low oestrogen levels. In overweight women with high oestrogen levels, the OCP will protect the uterus from cancer.

A tailor-made OCP can be designed to reduce excessive levels of male hormones in the woman with amenorrhoea associated with acne and facial hair.

If pregnancy is desired, it is necessary to stimulate ovulation with fertility drugs such as clomiphene or gonadotrophin drugs. These drugs should be given by a specialist gynaecologist.

CHAPTER 4

HORMONAL HEADACHES

During my practice of medicine I have seen countless women who complain that around the time of menstrual bleeding they are plagued with horrible headaches. These headaches may occur in the several days preceding the onset of the menstrual flow, during menstruation or when it ceases. They can also occur around ovulation. We call these headaches "hormonal" in type as during these times the blood level of the hormone oestrogen falls. (See Diagram 7).

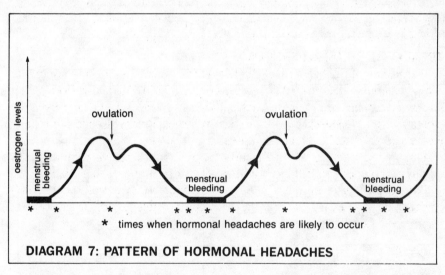

DIAGRAM 7: PATTERN OF HORMONAL HEADACHES

Every woman suffering with regular headaches should keep a menstrual and headache calendar to illustrate a possible hormonal link. If hormones are the trigger factor, a six-month calendar record will demonstrate the headache pattern. (See Maria's Calendar, Page 48).

The hormonal pattern of these headaches can change as a woman gets older, after childbirth, after hysterectomy or after surgical sterilization when the tubes are tied (tubal ligation). These factors may be associated with an overall decrease in the production of oestrogen from the ovaries when the usual cyclical drop in blood oestrogen becomes more extreme causing the headaches to be more frequent, more severe and to last longer.

MARIA'S CHART

	September	October	November	December
1	H			
2				
3		H		
4			H	
5				H
6				
7				
8				
9				
10				
11				
12				
13				
14	H			
15	M H	H		
16	M	H		
17	M H	M H	H	
18	M	M	M H	
19	M	M	M	H
20	H	M H	M H	M H
21		M	M H	M
22		H	M H	M H
23		H	H	M
24				M
25				
26				
27				
28				
29				
30				
31				

CODE: M = menstrual bleeding
     H = headache
Maria has a 5 day bleeding cycle every 32 days.
Ovulation occurs 14 days before menstrual bleeding starts.

One woman, aged 50, who came to see me complained of anxiety and depression and a migraine headache every second day. She said she'd been like this for twenty years ever since the removal of her uterus and ovaries at the age of 30. Yes, you guessed it, she had never received any Hormone Replacement Therapy. Thankfully, she had the common sense to avoid taking painkillers for her chronic headaches or she may very well have needed dialysis for analgesic induced kidney disease. She had resorted to taking ergotamine tablets daily to try to constrict the throbbing swollen blood vessels in her head but this made her nauseated and caused her hands and feet to be blue and cold. She felt sexless, miserable and trapped in the body of a woman older than her years.

After receiving natural oestrogen in the form of an implant she blossomed in a matter of four weeks into a serene, happy and attractive woman and I discovered that she had a delightful personality buried under all that pain. Her headaches became a rare event and she coped eminently well with far greater family stresses than ever before.

There were several reasons why she had taken so long to find relief. Firstly, her doctor had not recognised that migraine is often exacerbated by oestrogen deficiency and secondly, after she had been told that, "You have to learn to live with it", she felt guilty about complaining to doctors and was not sufficiently assertive in her pursuit of relief.

Why Do Hormones Cause Headaches?

The reason why a drop in blood oestrogen levels causes our head to ache is not fully understood. Oestrogen is a steroid hormone and, as such, probably exerts an anti-inflammatory effect upon our musculoskeletal tissues and a stabilising effect upon the blood vessels. It is logical that when blood oestrogen levels fall, this could trigger off an inflammatory and destabilising effect upon the blood vessels and musculoskeletal tissues in the head. This is experienced as a throbbing pain as the blood vessels constrict and then dilate excessively. We call this a "vascular headache" and if the disturbance to the brain's circulation is severe, a typical migraine headache may develop.

Someone who suffers with regular migraine is known as a "migraineur". True migraine may be associated with visual disturbances and vomiting and may last for 24 to 48 hours unless treatment is given. Women with hormonal headaches will often complain that the bones and muscles in their head and face are aching and tender to touch and in these cases a therapeutic massage on the tender trigger points can be helpful. Hormonal headaches may be associated with general body aches and pains, fatigue and depression which reflects the low levels of oestrogen at this time.

The Social Effects of Headaches

By charting the timing of headaches with hormonal fluctuations and menstrual bleeding, they may become predictable. Sufferers plan their professional and social lives around the headache times. It is particularly difficult for women with young children who lack a family support network as they often find it impossible to rest. The 20th-century career woman who needs to be performing at top level may find it difficult to compete when functional disorders associated with "hormones" or "menstruation" are still often wrongly minimised as "psychosomatic". This typical super-achiever and perfectionist will try to battle on not admitting to her peers that she is unwell with a cyclical vulnerability that could make her less productive than a man.

TREATMENT OF HORMONAL HEADACHES

Women who find that hormonal headaches can be alleviated and prevented feel a relief akin to being "sprung" from prison. If you refresh your memory with our graph in Diagram 7, it becomes obvious that if we can prevent the blood oestrogen levels from falling, we can stop the trigger factor for a hormonal headache. The oestrogen can be given in several ways and, most importantly, it needs to be given **every day** to prevent blood oestrogen levels from falling.

The Oral Contraceptive Pill

Many migraine/vascular headache sufferers are unable to tolerate the oral contraceptive pill (OCP) as it can aggravate the frequency and severity of migraines or occasionally bring them on for the first time, while others find that the OCP does indeed effectively reduce hormonal-vascular type headaches. So the OCP can be unpredictable in its effect on headaches and it can be necessary to simply try it and see how you go, although severe migraine sufferers should avoid the OCP. The mini pill or "progesterone only pill" is an exception and is usually well tolerated by migraineurs. If the headache occurs only during menstruation in a woman on the OCP, it is necessary to give a low dose of oestrogen during the seven-day pill break (or seven days of sugar pills) between pill cycles. This could be tablets of ethinyl oestradiol 10mcg daily, or an oestrogen patch given during the seven day break and your local doctor could prescribe this.

Some women will be unable to tolerate any reduction of their oestrogen dose, and the 10mcg of ethinyl oestradiol given daily during the seven-day pill break will not prevent the headaches.

In such cases, a tailor-made OCP can be tried giving ethinyl oestradiol 50mcg daily every day, and a progestogen such as norethisterone given for fifteen days every month to bring on a regular menstrual bleed and regulate the cycle. There are many possible variations of tailor-made oral contraceptive pills.

The OCP should be stopped immediately if it causes migraines associated with visual disturbances such as blurred vision, flashing lights or golden lights, or neurological problems such as clumsiness, weakness, numbness, pins and needles in the limbs. In such cases the risk of a stroke (brain haemorrhage) is increased, especially in women over the age of 35 who smoke.

Natural Oestrogen

In women not requiring oral contraception, the natural forms of oestrogen can be given with the aim of maintaining constant oestrogen blood levels. If you have had a hysterectomy, this is a simple matter and natural oestrogen can be given in the form of daily tablets, the oestrogen patch, fortnightly injections or a six-monthly implant of oestradiol.

Life is a bit more complicated for those among us who still have a uterus, in which case it is necessary to balance oestrogen with some type of progestogen. One possibility is to take the tablet of natural oestrogen every day without a break and along with this take a progestogen such as Provera 5mg to 10mg for fourteen days every month. The Provera given in this cyclical fashion will bring on a regular menstrual bleed.

If headaches still occur at the time of menstruation, it is then possible to avoid menstruation altogether by taking both progestogen and natural oestrogen every day. This practice has been found to be effective and safe.

I often emphasise, "Every woman is an individual" and what works for one woman may not work for another. This is definitely true when it comes to hormone therapy and there will be a significant percentage of women who find that oral oestrogen (tablet forms) causes their headaches to worsen. In such cases, it may be worthwhile to withdraw all hormone therapy for three to six months and observe what happens to the headaches during a woman's own natural menstrual cycle. If the headaches still persist on a cyclical basis, it is then time to try oestrogen replacement in a different form. Presently, one has the choice of an oestrogen implant, oestrogen injections and oestrogen patches which supply oestrogen in the natural form of oestradiol. The implant can be inserted every six to twelve months or the injection administered into the muscle of the buttocks every one to two weeks. The oestrogen patch is worn every day and replaced every third day with a new patch.

If you still have a uterus, progestrone will also need to be given for fourteen days every month to regulate the bleeding cycle. Occasionally, the synthetic progestrone tablets will produce undesirable side effects and induce a pre-menstrual syndrome-like state with a recurrence of the headaches. In such cases, a neutral progestrone may be given once a month in the form of a "Prolution Depot" injection into the buttocks. Alternatively, you may use natural progesterone lozenges (troches) during the fourteen premenstrual days. For availability call 02 9387 3205.

The observation that some women cannot tolerate oral forms of oestrogen and progesterone is common enough and is an interesting phenomenon. Many of this group of women will feel well taking oestrogen if it is given as injections, implants, patches or creams. We call these non-oral forms of oestrogen "parenteral oestrogen". Oestrogen given in this way is absorbed directly into the blood circulation and bypasses the liver thus having less effect on the function of the liver. Many migraineurs find that they feel "liverish" during their headache attacks with nausea and vomiting or they complain that fatty or rich foods strain their liver and gall bladder and bring on a headache. These migraineurs need to reduce stress upon their livers and this is why parenteral oestrogen can be preferable to oral oestrogen. For similar liverish reasons, migraineurs are wise to avoid all but the smallest amounts of alcohol and consume a liver-friendly diet. This diet is abundant in fresh vegetables and fruits, grains, legumes, seeds, cereals and fish. Fatty or fried foods and foods containing tyramine (red wine, beer, chocolate, lima and Italian beans, mature cheeses, chicken liver, raisins, avocados, plums) are best avoided. Also, avoid salty foods and monosodium glutamate.

All migraineurs should endeavour to increase their daily water intake to around two to three litres, preferably bottled spring water or purified water. This simple measure alone can greatly reduce the frequency of headaches. I have found that nutritional supplements of evening primrose oil 3000mg daily, antioxidant vitamins and the minerals zinc, calcium and magnesium often produce a worthwhile improvement in chronic headache sufferers.

TREATMENT OF AN ACUTE MIGRAINE

The key to success with an acute migraine lies in striking the attack on the head, so to speak, with measures being taken at the first hint of the migraine's onslaught.

Drug Approach

Preparations containing the drug ergotamine can be excellent in stopping the development of a migraine as they prevent the blood vessels from swelling and throbbing. Ergotamine must be taken at the first sign of the migraine and is versatile being available as tablets, injections or suppositories. If ergotamine causes nausea, simply reduce the dosage or take it in suppository form. Some women flnd that one-half to one-third of a suppository of an ergotamine preparation such as Cafergot is enough to do the trick.

Ergotamine should be taken together with a painkiller such as Aspalgin (aspirin + codeine) or Mersyndol. A tablet or suppository to stop nausea and vomiting may be essential, e.g., Stemetil or Maxalon. Some women find the new drug called Sumatriptan highly effective in stopping migraine.

Other Strategies

Non-drug approaches for the early stages of an acute migraine or cluster headache may be effective. I have had success giving intravenous vitamin C in one litre of a mineral solution and in cases of dehydration 2 litres intravenously may be required. Clinical studies have shown that the inhalation of medical oxygen via a face mask can be up to 80% effective in relieving a migraine or cluster headache.

You can ask your local doctor about the availability of medical oxygen. He may have a cylinder in his surgery or may be able to fill in the necessary paperwork so that you can hire a cylinder of oxygen for use in your own home.

HEADACHES AND PREGNANCY

The vast majority of migraineurs are free of headaches after the first six weeks of pregnancy because of the very high levels of oestrogen circulating in their bodies. During pregnancy, levels of the hormone progesterone are also very high and this causes relaxation of all the ligaments in the pelvis, joints and spine. Occasionally, the ligaments in the neck relax excessively causing the head to be unduly mobile upon the neck. This may result in unaccustomed headaches and even migraines especially in the mornings as the head may have twisted in relation to the neck during sleep.

This happened to a friend of mine who suffered terrible migraines for the first time in her life during her first pregnancy. She consulted many doctors to no avail and finally came across a chiropractor who told her to wear a firm foam rubber collar (cervical collar) to support her neck during sleep. From that point on she never had a morning migraine which was indeed fortunate as she has had three more children. Cervical collars can be purchased from your local pharmacy.

CHAPTER 5

POSTNATAL DEPRESSION

Depression after childbirth, known as postnatal depression is a common problem in modern society affecting between 10% to 40% of young mothers. It may also be referred to as post-partum or puerperal depression and the most important thing for women to realise is that, if it is correctly diagnosed, it can be cured. Postnatal depression may rear its ugly head any time during the first year after the baby's birth and inflict itself upon the most unsuspecting and unlikely candidates. It is just as likely to occur in women who have spent years in infertility clinics trying desperately to have a baby as it is in those women whose well ordered lives have been interrupted with an unwanted pregnancy.

There are three types of postnatal mood disorders which are distinct in their features and require different treatment. It is helpful to look at the features of these three different types:

The Maternity Blues

This is sometimes called the "post-partum blues" or "third day blues" and is just about as common as "lovers blues", so much so that some clever guitarist should write a 12-bar blues song to play over the radio to offer solace to these tearful new mothers. Postnatal wards in women's hospitals are sometimes called the "weeping wards" as at any one time about 50% to 80% of its inpatients will be feeling overly emotional and excessively tearful.

Thankfully, maternity blues don't last too long and are generally not severe, followed by a spontaneous return to a normal, happy, emotional state about 14 days after childbirth. This transient change in the emotional personality does not require any medication and will pass with support, rest and reassurance.

If the birth has been prolonged or difficult, the new mother is often physically and mentally drained, feeling very anxious that she will not cope with the baby's needs and this can precipitate anxious and tearful moments as can breastfeeding problems if they are not handled tactfully and patiently.

The nursery and medical staff should take great pains to try and accommodate the wishes of the new mother regarding the way she wants to spend the first few postnatal days with her baby as things that may appear tiny

DIAGRAM 8: HORMONAL CHANGES IN
PREGNANCY AND POSTNATAL PERIOD

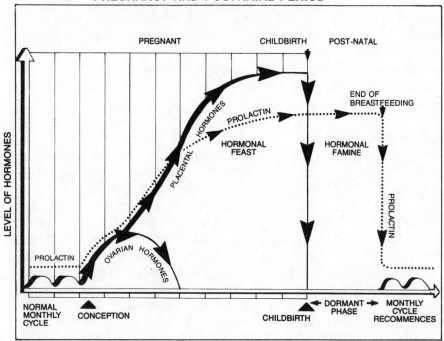

and inconsequential to others may seem vitally important to her and her relationship with her husband and baby. Doctors and nurses must realise that a new mother is vulnerable, dependent and often highly emotional, in need of support and sensitivity from those looking after her.

I remember an older mother coming to see me nine months after the birth of her second child, complaining of depression, anxiety and insomnia. She told me that she was haunted by the memory of the suturing of her episiotomy (vaginal cut) immediately after the birth of her baby. Her own obstetrician had been unavailable and his locum doctor had been called in at 3 a.m. to do the stitching. This doctor had complained bitterly about his disturbed sleep and had joked with the nursing staff about his drunken weekend. He had refused to allow the mother to cuddle and breastfeed the baby immediately before he began stitching the vaginal tear which had taken a full forty minutes. This woman found the doctor and staff totally insensitive and had longed for a quiet romantic twenty minutes with her baby immediately after birth. This patient was very angry and resentful and being unable to express this to the doctor she had turned it inside upon herself resulting in depression.

The sudden hormonal withdrawal during the first 24 hours after birth (See Diagram 8) is partly responsible for the third-day blues and may also cause a hormonal migraine, an increase in general aches and pains and, occasionally, in susceptible women, a flair up of arthritis, auto immune disorders or an asthma attack. These physical discomforts require specific treatment as they only add to the feelings of vulnerability and dependency in these early postnatal days.

Puerperal Psychosis

The second type of postnatal mood disorder is called puerperal psychosis and is a severe mental imbalance that needs urgent medical treatment. This type is vastly different to the common and mild maternity blues and, thankfully, is relatively rare occurring in only two to three per thousand births.

Puerperal psychosis usually has a sudden and dramatic onset, manifesting within the first two to three weeks after childbirth and may occur as early as several hours after birth. It produces a total change in the mental state with the thoughts and emotions becoming jumbled, frenzied, confused and irrational. The helpless victim of this psychosis becomes totally out of touch with reality being tormented and preoccupied with weird thoughts that may cause her to behave in an agitated and paranoid manner. She may be subject to hallucinations of sight and smell, seeing and hearing voices and things that are not present and imagining that she or her baby are in imminent and grave danger. Understandably, she may become disorientated and unable to sleep, eat or care for her child.

Christine, a 31-year-old single mother had had a normal pregnancy and easy vaginal delivery of a healthy baby and all seemed well as I wished her good night after checking her baby. The next morning when I arrived at her bedside, she had become a different person with an agitated and worried look upon her face. She insisted that the nurses had put a spell on her baby that made him susceptible to evil spirits and that her breast milk was poisonous. She wanted to purify the baby by putting him on a fast and giving him a bath in holy water. She asked me to urgently find a priest to exorcise the spirit out of her son with a cross and holy bible. Christine was continuously distracted by loud voices although in reality her ward was quiet and almost empty and she complained that her breast milk smelt rotten and unwholesome.

The nursing staff were unable to restrain or control this large powerful woman and an urgent injection of tranquillising medication was required. It was nine months before Christine was able to care for her baby without constant supervision.

The most dangerous aspect of post-partum psychosis is that a sufferer may have compulsions or obsessions to harm herself or her baby and suicide and infanticide are not rare in this disorder. One psychotic woman became so obsessed with the long shape of her baby's head that she was found trying to hammer it back into a rounder shape. Every year a case of severe puerperal psychosis tragically makes the newspaper headlines and we read that:

"Mother jumped out of hospital window with her baby"

"Mother stabs three children"

"Child suffocated by distraught mother"

"Two children and mother asphyxiated with car exhaust".

These tragedies should not occur and if society, families and professionals were more aware of the early stages of post-partum psychosis, life-saving emergency treatment could be given. It is incredible to think that Governments spend billions of dollars trying to cure AIDS, cancer and heart disease and yet post-partum psychosis which is easier to prevent and cure than these diseases, receives very little funding or attention and these tragedies continue.

Obviously, these women need 24-hour observation in a security hospital environment and major tranquillising drugs. The mother cannot be left alone with the baby under any circumstances even in the safety of a mother and baby unit within the hospital or mothercraft centre.

Post-partum psychosis requires powerful tranquillising drugs and when the mother is discharged from hospital care her behaviour and emotional state is still influenced by these drugs so that she is usually slow and unable to care for her baby by herself. Generally, she would take many months to several years for complete recovery, although hormonal therapy with natural progesterone may shorten her illness.

She, or her family, should be instructed to keep a menstrual calendar to check for pre-menstrual deteriorations in her mental state and once she is stable an attempt can be made to reduce her tranquillisers. She may require extra progesterone to control pre-menstrual exacerbations of her psychosis.

Postnatal Depression

This illness falls in between the maternity blues and post-partum psychosis being more severe than the former and less incapacitating and destructive than the latter. Postnatal depression is really a mixed bag of problems that varies in the type of symptoms, their severity and duration. Postnatal depression is very common as 10% to 40% of women are affected. The symptoms of postnatal depression may start any time in the 12 months after birth. Some people do not realise this so postnatal depression may not be recognised for what it is, especially if it begins as long as 6 months after childbirth. Most commonly it lasts for several months but up to one in five women with postnatal depression are still feeling unwell 12 months after the birth.

What Are the Symptoms of Postnatal Depression?

A woman may have some or all of the following:-

1. Psychological Symptoms

Depression, sadness, irritability, anxiety, loss of confidence, excessive worrying, panic attacks, feelings of unworthiness, anger, resentment, guilt, irrational fears, obsessions, excessive sleepiness or inability to sleep, emotional desolation with lack of feeling for the baby, rejection of the baby or excessive attachment to the baby, feeling spaced out, confusion, reduced intellectual and mental function, preoccupation with death, suicidal thoughts and wishes and desires to harm the baby.

2. Physical Symptoms

Light-headed feelings, low blood sugar, muscle aches and pains with flu-like feelings, headaches, increased or decreased appetite or thirst, eating binges with sugar and junk foods, increased or decreased weight, constipation and extreme exhaustion.

Some mothers are too ashamed and feel too guilty to accept or complain that they are depressed and convert their emotional stress into physical symptoms. For instance, a young mother with masked depression may pay frequent visits to her doctor for minor physical complaints such as fatigue, or a crying colicky or vomiting baby. If the doctor cannot find any physical signs of abnormality he should look deeper as the mother may be desperate for emotional help but cannot ask as she does not want to be stigmatised as an inadequate mother.

It is vital that women with postnatal depression receive early and adequate treatment because if it is allowed to progress it may have a devastating effect upon the family and produce marital conflict and a deterioration in the relationship between the depressed mother and her baby. The babies of depressed mothers are more likely to suffer with feeding and sleeping difficulties and develop mental problems. Professor of psychiatry at Monash University, Professor Bruce Tong, has found that such babies may become either emotionally distant and detached from their mothers or more clinging and demanding and unable to be soothed. Professor Tong found that if the depression continued for twelve months the baby may become irritable with reduced concentration or show less interest in surrounding activities than the babies of non-depressed mothers. If the depression should become deeper, a mother could get to the stage of not coping and may be at risk of harming the baby. She may shake or spank the baby excessively or feel like throwing it on the floor. The guilty feelings engendered by this behaviour make it even more difficult for her to ask for help. A vicious circle develops and it is easy for social isolation to occur.

3. Sexuality and Postnatal Depression

Women with postnatal depression often have a loss of interest in sex and may even become sexually frigid to the point of being annoyed or repulsed by the advances of their partner. This may be due to a combination of their loss of sex hormones, physical exhaustion, side effects from anti-depressant medication or inadequate contraception, especially if the birth has been painful or traumatic.

Lindy had given birth to a bouncing baby boy in February and all was going well until postnatal depression insidiously set in during the following May. She stopped breastfeeding and her first menstruation which was heralded by severe pre-menstrual syndrome arrived in June. She felt some relief after her menstruation began, although the following months were distressful as she was exhausted and totally disinterested in sex which made her husband irritable and cranky. In September she approached her doctor as she was worried about depression, sexual frigidity, absent periods and continuing milk from her breast even though she had stopped breastfeeding in May.

The presence of inappropriate breast milk in the absence of breastfeeding is called galactorrhoea and is often associated with an excessive production of the lactation hormone called "Prolactin" from the pituitary gland.

Lindy's doctor told her that her "menstrual clock" situated in the hypothalamus (See Page 20) was not working properly and when he measured the blood level of the hormone prolactin it was too high. Once he had ruled out the possibility of a pituitary tumour he started Lindy on a course of Bromocriptine (Parlodel) tablets to reduce her prolactin levels to normal.

If prolactin levels are too high, the ovaries remain in a dormant state and do not produce the female sex hormones oestrogen and progesterone and so regular menstruation does not occur. This is why full-time regular breastfeeding acts as a good contraceptive especially in Third World countries.

Lindy took the Bromocriptine tablets for eight weeks and, once her prolactin levels came down, her breast milk dried up, her menstruation returned and she began once more to feel sexually alive.

Prolactin is not the only hormone that may be out of balance postnatally and if you are suffering with loss of libido or sexual difficulties during your first postnatal year, it is wise to have a blood test to check your levels of the sex steroid hormones, oestrogen and testosterone as these are largely responsible for creating sexual desire. Also, ask your doctor to check the levels of free testosterone as it is the free or unbound component of testosterone that is active in your body. The best measure of free male hormones is the "free androgen index" or F.A.I. which is easily measured in a simple blood test and this is often very low in women with poor libido or sexual frigidity.

Some women find that the combined oral contraceptive pill is not suiting them postnatally as it may greatly reduce sexual desire as well as cause depression to persist. In such cases you may try a progesterone only contraceptive pill also known as a "mini pill" and if this does not improve matters, consider condoms or a vaginal diaphragm.

4. Physical Exhaustion

During the first six months after childbirth women may suffer with fatigue and lethargy, craving sleep and unable to get through the routine chores. If blood loss at birth was excessive, iron deficiency is common and, especially if breastfeeding, the body's iron stores quickly become depleted if supplemental iron is not given. If ordinary iron supplements cause constipation, I suggest you try an organic iron supplement such as "hemofactor" which should be taken in a dose of two tablets three times daily on an empty stomach with citrus fruit or vitamin C to aid absorption.

Other mineral deficiencies are not uncommon at this time and supplements of calcium, zinc, magnesium and potassium can be a wonderful aid to boost flagging energy reserves. Magnesium and potassium can be found together in a tablet called "K-Mag" available from pharmacies.

Your body is going through enormous physiological changes and in the first six postnatal weeks the blood volume diminishes and the uterus shrinks back to its non-pregnant size. If you are breastfeeding particularly in a hot climate, dehydration may cause profound exhaustion, and you should drink at least three litres of fluid daily in the form of purified water and/or raw vegetable juices.

If you find that your skin and hair become very dry and your metabolism slows down, ask your doctor to check the function of your thyroid gland as it may have become temporarily under-active. The thyroid gland can be helped along with kelp, spirulina and macrobiotic seaweed preparations and very occasionally it may be necessary to give a course of thyroid hormone tablets.

Some women who have been subjected to excessive and continuous stress postnatally may find that the cause of their fatigue is a temporary underactivity of their adrenal glands known as **"adrenal exhaustion"**. This may also occur after excessive blood loss at the time of birth.

Margaret's Story

Margaret had lost nearly a litre of blood from a tear of her cervix during the rapid vaginal birth of her daughter. Despite a blood transfusion she still felt exhausted four months after birth and complained that she had lost all her old energy. She felt dizzy and light-headed and continually craved sugar and carbohydrates.

I found that Margaret's blood pressure and blood sugar level were very low and that her blood cortisone levels were at the lower limit of normal in both the mornings and evenings.

The adrenal glands produce the hormone cortisone and other hormones involved in the control of blood sugar levels and blood pressure.

Margaret was not anaemic as she was on iron supplements. I diagnosed "adrenal exhaustion" which I reassured her would recover with rest and time. To speed up the adrenal recovery, I prescribed vitamin C with bioflavonoids 4000 mg daily and vitamin E 500 international units daily. To stabilise her blood sugar level, I prescribed amino acid complex containing all of the eight essential amino acids and a tablet called "Sucro" that contains B complex vitamins and synergistic minerals such as chromium, manganese and zinc. Margaret took the amino acids and sucro tablets with every meal and was encouraged to eat small frequent meals containing protein, complex carbohydrate and raw fruit and vegetables.

First-class protein and complex carbohydrates can be obtained by combining three of the following — grains, nuts, seeds and legumes at one meal. Other good sources of first class protein are lean meats, fish, seafoods, chicken, eggs and low-fat dairy products.

After six weeks on her new diet and supplements Margaret regained her old vitality. Her blood sugar and cortisone levels increased and she was delighted that she had easily shed 3kg of surplus fat now that she no longer binged on chocolate and cookies.

Hormonal Changes in Pregnancy

In the non-pregnant woman, the regular monthly menstrual cycle is controlled by the hormonal rhythm regulator or "hormonal clock" situated in the area of the brain called the hypothalamus. (See Diagram 4 on Page 20). Once conception occurs, around day 14 of the menstrual cycle, the production of oestrogen and progesterone from the ovaries increases to higher levels than those found in a non-pregnant woman. (See Diagram 8 on Page 55). The early surge of ovarian hormones immediately after conception may induce headaches, nausea, fatigue and sore breasts even before the next period is missed. Some women may feel quite different and be sure that they are pregnant within several days after conception.

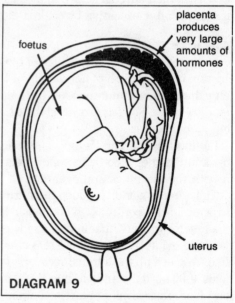

placenta produces very large amounts of hormones

foetus

uterus

DIAGRAM 9

In early pregnancy, hormonal control is taken over by the placenta and foetus and the "Hormonal clock" in the hypothalamus becomes inactive until menstruation returns after childbirth. The cells surrounding the tiny embryo pump out the unique pregnancy hormone called "human chorionic gonadotrophin" (HCG) which stimulates the ovaries to greatly increase their production of oestrogen and progesterone. During the first eight weeks of pregnancy, oestrogen and progesterone are mainly produced by the ovary, but after this time the placenta becomes dominant and behaves like a huge endocrine gland gradually increasing its manufacture of oestrogen and progesterone to enormous levels (See Diagrams 8 and 9.) The placenta is very efficient and produces progesterone levels 50 to 300 times higher and oestrogen levels 10 to 50 times higher than the maximum levels found during a normal non-pregnant menstrual cycle. During pregnancy the pituitary gland produces large quantities of Prolactin hormone and the adrenal glands double their output of cortisone. Thus, during pregnancy we could say that women enjoy a "hormonal feast" and this is why most women feel so well mentally and physically during pregnancy. One of my patients who has premenstrual syndrome commented that during pregnancy she feels like Superwoman and rediscovers the woman she is meant to be. She made me laugh when she told me that she was considering applying for a full-time job as a surrogate mother.

The Hormonal Drama of Childbirth

Within hours after the delivery of the baby and placenta, there is a large and precipitous fall in the levels of the sex hormones so that only tiny amounts of these hormones are found in the mother's body. What has taken nine months to develop is suddenly withdrawn and a woman passes from a "hormonal feast" to a "hormonal famine" in a matter of several hours. Progesterone disappears completely by the seventh day after birth and oestrogen levels out at very low amounts in the same time span. Synonymous with this, the pituitary gland pumps out large amounts of Prolactin to produce lactation and the ovaries enter into a dormant or resting phase. (See Diagram 8.) The high levels of Prolactin ensure that the ovary remains unresponsive and dormant and thus the levels of the ovarian sex hormones oestrogen and progesterone remain very low until a woman decides to stop breastfeeding and Prolactin levels subsequently return to normal. Thus, the length of the dormant phase of the ovaries varies from several weeks to several years depending upon the duration of breastfeeding and high Prolactin levels. During the dormant postnatal phase of the ovaries, the menstrual clock in the hypothalamus is switched off and remains so until menstruation returns.

The hypothalamus also regulates mood, sleep, appetite and day/night body rhythms. Because these basic body functions are often disturbed in women with postnatal depression, many experts believe that the hypothalamic control centres may be at fault.

When one understands the precipitous hormonal drama of childbirth it is easy to understand that these hormonal changes can initiate maternity blues, post-partum psychosis or postnatal depression. Indeed, it is truly amazing that most women come through these hormonal upheavals without complaining and they should be commended and praised for this.

The Treatment of Postnatal Depression

It is true to say that sometimes the treatment of postnatal depression appears somewhat confused with different doctors having very different approaches to helping a woman with depression after childbirth. This is because the treatment of postnatal depression falls in between the three different medical specialities of obstetrics, psychiatry and endocrinology. This is of little comfort to the depressed and ailing woman who only wishes to find the quickest and safest way out of her desolation.

It is reassuring to know that postnatal depression can be completely cured provided it is recognised and treated early after birth. Furthermore, postnatal depression can be prevented from reccurring after subsequent pregnancies, provided once again treatment is given immediately after birth. There are many women who do not realise this and are too frightened to have further children. Dr. Katharina Dalton has found that without preventative treatment the chance of postnatal depression recurring after subsequent births is 2 out of 3. (Reference 1.)

HORMONAL TREATMENT

Progesterone

Treatment of postnatal depression with natural progesterone is rather controversial among the experts. However, large studies of women with postnatal depression in the UK conducted by Dr. Dalton (Reference 1) have found injections and suppositories/pessaries of progesterone to be fairly successful.

Dalton found that the natural recurrence rate of 2 in 3 for postnatal depression could be reduced to less than 1 in 10 if progesterone was given immediately after childbirth. Dalton believes that after birth the precipitous fall in progesterone to negligible levels initiates the depression, and thus if progesterone injections are given to reduce this fall, the depression will be lessened. She recommends that progesterone is given as an intra-muscular injection in a dose of 100mg daily for the first seven days after birth. In Australia, natural progesterone injections are only available in the form of Proluton 25mg ampoules. Thus, you would need four of these 25mg ampoules to be drawn up into one syringe which could be injected deeply into the buttocks once a day for seven days. The first of these progesterone injections must be given at the completion of birth before the symptoms of postnatal depression begin and Dalton says that the anti-depressant effect of this progesterone is greatly lessened if the injections are delayed until symptoms are present.

Natural progesterone is very safe, does not interfere with breastfeeding and does not affect the new-born babe, but its main drawback is its expense. **For information on the availability of progesterone see the Appendix on pages 144-145.**

After the first seven postnatal days, the progesterone injections are replaced with progesterone vaginal pessaries or rectal suppositories which are given in a dose of 2, 200mg pessaries twice daily providing a total daily progesterone dose of 800mg. These pessaries/suppositories are continued until the menstrual periods return, so that breastfeeding mothers may need to continue them for many months. Once improvement has occurred, the number of progesterone pessaries can be gradually reduced down to 1 or 2 daily.

Other Hormones

For postnatal depression in older women, or if it is associated with loss of libido and marital discord, the temporary use of natural oestrogen and testosterone can be very effective in elevating the mood and energy levels and in restoring sexual desire and pleasure. Oestrogen should not be given during the first two weeks after childbirth as there is an increased risk of thrombosis (blood clots) at this time. Furthermore, oestrogen and/or testosterone cannot be used in breastfeeding women as they reduce the milk supply and these hormones can adversely affect the baby. Oestrogen and/or testosterone can be started two weeks after birth in women who do not want to breastfeed and who are active and ambulant. Adequate contraception in the form of the progesterone only mini pill, a low dose contraceptive pill, condoms, vaginal diaphragm or an intra-uterine contraceptive device is necessary. If you decide to try natural oestrogen and testosterone to overcome your postnatal depression, I suggest you receive it in the form of Primodian injections which are given deeply into the buttocks at monthly intervals. Primodian injections should be continued until the depression disappears and, in general, three to four injections are necessary, although in milder cases only one injection is sufficient.

If the postnatal depression returns in a severe form after stopping the Primodian injections, you may want to consider the option of having an implant of natural oestrogen, or natural oestrogen and testosterone which has a longer effect than the injections and should prevent the depression from returning.

Drug Treatments

Bromocriptine (Parlodel): This drug lowers the level of the pituitary hormone Prolactin and so smartly brings breastfeeding to an end. It may be tried in women with postnatal depression and poor libido who do not want to breastfeed. Parlodel will speed up the return of ovulation and menstruation and thus normal levels of oestrogen and progesterone will return in the monthly cyclical pattern. This should relieve depression and poor libido due to the very low levels of sex hormones found in the dormant phase of the postnatal period. (See Diagram 8 on Page 55).

Parlodel is taken as 1 or 2 tablets with food last thing at night, because if taken during the day or without food, it may produce headaches, nausea or dizziness.

Anti-Depressant Drugs: Some women with postnatal depression may need anti-depressant medication and we do not have a test that will tell us if your depression will respond to hormones, anti-depressants or if it will require both. Thus, patience is required from both the doctor and the patient and although a little trial and error may occur, effective relief is sure to be found.

Tricyclic Anti-Depressant Drugs: These drugs have been used for many years to treat all types of depression and are particularly effective if the depression is associated with anxiety, worried thoughts, excessive mental activity, reduced appetite and poor sleep. It is best to start with small doses as many women respond to these and it is possible to continue breastfeeding if you are only taking small to moderate doses of the tricyclic anti-depressant drugs. If your doctor finds it necessary to increase the dose of these drugs, do not be alarmed as this is only temporary and these drugs are very safe. Examples of tricyclic drugs are Trofranil, Sinequan, Prothiaden. **Monoamine Oxidase Inhibitors (MAOI):** These drugs prevent your enzymes from breaking down the brain's neuro-transmitters and in particular those called the biogenic amines which are powerful anti-depressants. Examples of the MAOI drugs are Parnate and Aurorix.

The Monoamine Oxidase Inhibitor drugs are powerful anti-depressants and may be very helpful for you if your postnatal depression is associated with a complete loss of energy, mental dullness, apathy and loss of interest in your family and surroundings. The advantages of the MAOI drugs are that they work quickly, do not cause drowsiness as a side effect and indeed they wake you up, so that they should be taken on awakening and no later than 3 pm and definitely not at night. The group of drugs known as serotonin reuptake inhibitors are excellent anti-depressants, examples of which are Prozac, Zoloft and Aropax. These drugs are often necessary for twelve months or more to really cure postnatal depression.

Stopping Medications

This should always be done gradually with small reductions in the dose being made in two-weekly or monthly steps. This applies if you are taking anti-depressant drugs or progesterone. The reduction should be made at the end of menstrual bleeding and not during the pre-menstrual phase.

Be Prepared

It is not wise to first consider postnatal depression once it has hit you. You and your family should discuss this possibility during pregnancy so that you are all able to recognise the first signs of this illness. If you have already suffered with a bout of postnatal depression, make sure that during your next pregnancy you discuss all your treatment options with your family, general practitioner and obstetrician while you are still objective about it. If progesterone injections may be necessary these can be pre-arranged by your general practitioner and obstetrician to be available for you at the hospital immediately after birth.

PSYCHOLOGY AND POSTNATAL DEPRESSION

This is a huge subject and it is not possible in a book about hormones to physically fit it all in. The reader is recommended to read the book *The New Mother Syndrome* by Carol Dix and published by Allen & Unwin to explore the psychological effects of having a baby.

I myself have never had children and so do not really feel qualified to tackle the psychological consequences that babies may provoke in our lives. I've left this to my sister Madeleine to tell you how she felt hormonally, mentally and emotionally after childbirth.

SURVIVING THE FIRST YEAR AFTER CHILDBIRTH

Being a woman is a fantastic gift. We have the opportunity to experience life growing within us, giving birth and then sustaining that new life and watching it grow. We become intrinsically linked with the process of the cycle of birth and death. Pretty amazing stuff! So who said it was going to be easy! As women, we are by nature intuitive and instinctive beings and our hormonal cycle is bound by the lunar phases which have great power over many of the processes of nature.

Surviving the changes that befall us during pregnancy and lactation is no menial task and one we are definitely not educated for. It is imperative that we trust our own intuition and believe in our own ability as every child is different and if we can only "tune in" to that child and trust and follow our instincts, it will all unfold as it is meant to do.

The most important thing is your attitude. Don't cling to ideas and concepts about how it is going to be or how it should be. You may feel great and have an angelic baby or you may feel terrible and have a screaming baby that never sleeps. Accept it and flow with it or life is going to be frustrating, bewildering and beset with negativity and unfulfilment. All the above is easy to say and difficult to achieve. I learnt from my first child to let go within the first week of our life together. What does 'let go' mean? It meant accepting that he was the kind of baby that never slept, breastfed every 1½ hours, screamed with colic and took more than I had to give.

What happened to my life? It became non-existent! My other two children were much easier to cope with, especially after having a first child like this. So, having accepted that he was an abominable baby, who has since grown into an amazing teenager, I had to work out how I was going to survive the first year.

I was very tired. Absolutely exhausted would be more truthful, frightened, vulnerable and full of self-doubt. None of my family had any idea how to cope with him, my husband included. His first thought at the time of birth was "That's very nice, but can we put it back in now!" So I bought a king-size bed and put him in between myself and my husband because when he woke at night I found it easy to put him on the breast and feed him lying down. We got a lot more sleep that way. In a word, I learnt very quickly how to totally surrender. He bathed with me or my husband and I bought a snugly

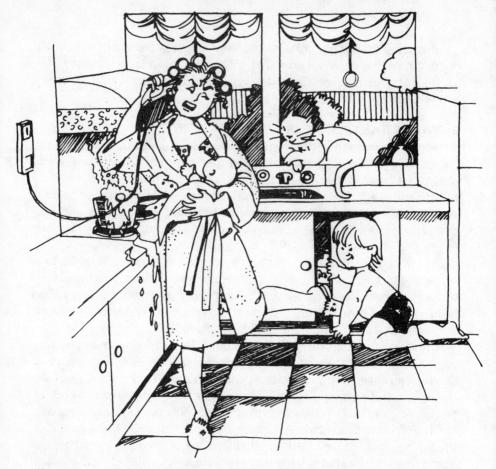

to carry him around in and life settled down a little. He became like an extra limb always hanging there somewhere.

Everyone tried to tell me I was doing the wrong thing, spoiling him and making a rod for my own back. I just trusted what we had going and then it became far more enjoyable.

Having no time left for yourself can be very awesome — a bit like a prison sentence. I mean washing your hair becomes a luxury and when one of your fantasies becomes sleeping eight hours through without interruption — you know you've got it bad.

Life becomes an endless saga of changing nappies, washing, cleaning, breastfeeding and just keeping baby happy. Ah! the joys of motherhood. One suffers from:

a) Looking in the mirror at the 5 kilograms you still have to lose. Just keep breastfeeding and it will go.

b) Isolation and lack of adult company. Your friends find it all a bit boring and it becomes difficult to get out of the house.

c) Total loss of your sexual identity. How can you feel sexy when you don't ever get to do anything that stimulates that part of your psyche.

d) Loss of personal achievements other than motherhood.

e) Loss of freedom. Will you ever be able to have a phone conversation without harassment again? What happened to those long baths and lazy lunches with friends?

f) Tiredness, anxiety over baby's health problems (of which there are many), stitches, sore nipples, mastitis, haemorrhoids, weakness. The list is endless.

g) Feeling alone, misunderstood and discontented.

All women feel some of the above and if they deny it, they must be numb or lying to themselves. It is natural to feel like this, our body's hormonal cycle is still in fluctuation and we had so many ideas and romantic notions that have no doubt taken a beating. I remember looking out the window and just waiting for my mother to arrive every morning after my third child was born, which she did, thank God for six weeks. We need somebody understanding to help us through this initial phase and we need our husbands to realise that if there is nothing left of ourselves for us, how can there be any left for them. We need support, not extra demands. With time, we reclaim our identity on all levels and what an incredible joy it is. It's like being re-born.

Being a mother has taught me the value of time and I have had to learn so many lessons about myself that I might otherwise have run away from. It is the greatest love you'll ever know and the greatest sacrifice you'll ever make. Where would the world be without relationships like grandmother to granddaughter, daughter to mother, mother to son. Remember, don't take yourself too seriously and don't expect too much of yourself. Take it day by day and trust in yourself totally because then all things become possible.

REFERENCE

1. Dalton K. *Depression after Childbirth*, Oxford University Press.

HELPFUL RESOURCES FOR POSTNATAL DEPRESSION

New South Wales

Postnatal Depression Kit — contains a video called "The baby's fine, but how are you?" combined with three booklets. Produced by St. Margarets Private Hospital — (02) 339-0460. Also from National and State Libraries.

Karitane Mother Craft Hospital — (02) 399 7111.

Tresillian Mother Craft Hospital — (02) 568 3633.

Postnatal Depression 24 hour help line — (02) 569 5400

Victoria

Mercy Maternity Hospital, mother and baby unit, outpatient and inpatient facilities — (03) 270 2222.

Monash Medical Centre, Assessment Clinic for Postnatal Depression — (03) 550 1111.

Queensland

Postnatal Depression Support Group, 27 Garoona Grove, Slacks Creek 4127. Sharon — (07) 209 2773. Jan — (07) 359 6293.

Royal Brisbane Hospital, mother and baby unit — (07) 253 8111.

Royal Women's Hospital — (07) 253-7833.

Extension Midwifery Services — (07) 253 7587.

Residential Centre, 184 St Pauls Terrace, Brisbane — (07) 252 8555.

Western Australia

Post Partum Depression Interest Association (PPDIA), 7 Camelia Court, Ferndale 6155. — (09) 451 3942.

King Edward Hospital, Department of Social Work — (09) 340 2222.

Northern Territory

Casuarina Community Health Centre, Casuarina Plaza, Cnr Trower Road and Vanderlin Drive, Casuarina 5792. — (089) 22 7301.

South Australia

Overcoming Postnatal Depression (OPND) PO Box 306 Daw Park 5041. — (08) 277 3340.

Child, Adolescent & Family Healh Services (CAFHS), 295 South Terrace, Adelaide 5000. 24 hour telephone advisory service (08) 236 0444.

Glenside Family Unit for Postnatal Depression and Psychosis, multi-disciplinary specialist team, 24 hour counselling. PO Box 17, Eastwood 5063. — (08) 372 1183.

CHAPTER 6

CONTRACEPTION – AND HOW IT CAN AFFECT YOUR HORMONES

The Oral Contraceptive Pill (OCP)

So far, this book has dealt with how your own hormones can affect you, and yet four out of every five western women in their mid-30s either takes, or has taken at some time, the Oral Contraceptive Pill (OCP) which suppresses their own sex hormones. The combined OCP contains synthetic oestrogen and progesterone which switch off the menstrual clock in the hypothalamus so that the ovaries do not receive a message to produce an egg, so ovulation does not occur and the ovaries do not produce their normal quota of natural oestrogen and progesterone.

The synthetic hormones comprising the various brands of oral contraceptive pills (OCPs) are primarily designed to prevent conception, but they may also exert both favourable and unfavourable effects upon a woman. In this chapter we shall explore these effects.

Today's modern low-dose OCP remains the most efficient and safest form of contraception. The triphasic OCPs (Triquilar or Triphasil), with the smallest amount of hormones, contain less hormones in one month's packet than one tablet of the original OCP designed thirty years ago!

To help you put the risk of the OCP into perspective, taking a relatively high dose OCP (by today's standards) is no more dangerous than going for a one-hour drive in your car. In the context of the fact that the combined oral contraceptive pill is the most effective form of contraception, its risks are offset by the risk to mother and child of unplanned and unwanted pregnancy or abortion.

THE DIFFERENT TYPES OF ORAL CONTRACEPTIVE PILL

The Combined Oral Contraceptive Pill (OCP)

This contains *both* oestrogen and progesterone in synthetic forms and in varying amounts, depending on the brand. The synthetic oestrogen used in the pill is ethinyl oestradiol and the synthetic progesterones are either norethisterone or levonorgestrel. Unfortunately, natural hormones as used in Hormone Replacement Therapy during the menopause, are not potent enough to prevent conception.

71

Of all the brands of combined OCPs available today, the triphasic OCP such as Triquilar comes closest to copying the natural menstrual cycle as it delivers varying amounts of hormones at different times in the menstrual cycle. This means that over one complete cycle, the total amount of hormone ingested is less than that from an oral contraceptive pill where the amount of hormone delivered is the same every day.

The Progesterone Only Pill

The Progesterone Only Pill (POP) is also referred to as the "mini pill". It contains only one hormone in the form of synthetic progesterone and does not contain oestrogen which is the other sex hormone. Commonly prescribed brands of the POP are Micronor or Microlut. Because the POP contains such a small amount of hormone, it must be taken every day, at the same time each day and without any breaks. It needs to be taken at least three hours before sexual intercourse, so that if you have sex later at night, you would be safe to take it around 6 pm each day. The POP provides such a low hormone dose that it causes only very small changes in your metabolism and thus does not cause any of the potentially serious side effects (such as blood clots, strokes or high blood pressure) occasionally associated with the combined OCP. The POP does not increase your risk of cardiovascular disease or cancer.

Because of its safety, the POP is an ideal contraceptive for women over 45 who are worried that the combined OCP may increase their chances of cardiovascular disease. Women over 35 who smoke, diabetics, migraine sufferers and women who get side effects from the combined OCP are also good candidates for the POP. (See Table 4 on Page 79). The POP is a suitable and safe contraceptive for breastfeeding women and women unable to take oestrogen for medical reasons such as liver disease, blood clots or high blood pressure.

The POP has a pregnancy rate of around 4% and is not quite as reliable as the combined OCP which has a failure rate of around 1%. The POP is more suited to older women or breastfeeding mothers whose fertility is less than that of younger or non-lactating women who may fear the 4% failure rate is unacceptable.

The mini pill is safe and generally well tolerated although one in four women get annoying irregular menstruation and breakthrough bleeding. This may be too problematic for sportive, outdoor women who like to control their menstrual cycle. Other women who should avoid the POP are those with a history of ectopic pregnancy, or pelvic inflammatory disease as the POP may increase your chances of ectopic pregnancy. An ectopic pregnancy is one occurring outside the uterus, usually in the uterine tubes.

How A Combined Oral Contraceptive Pill (OCP) Can Help You

Many women think that the only benefit of the combined OCP is the reliable protection against unwanted pregnancy and yet it may also confer other benefits and may be prescribed to help women with various gynaecological and hormonal problems. Let us take a look at some of the other effects of this pill upon your body.

1. Your menstrual bleeding will usually be controlled and regular. If you prefer to miss a period because of some special event, this is easy to plan simply by skipping the usual seven day break (or substitute sugar pills) between pill packets. In the vast majority of women on the combined OCP, menstrual bleeding becomes lighter and less painful and a complete relief of period cramps may often be obtained.

2. Your chances of pelvic infection from certain bacteria (such as gonorrhoea) may be less, although this does not apply to all pelvic infections and, in particular, the pill does not reduce your chances of infection with chlamydia. (See Reference 1).

3. Your chances of forming cysts on your ovaries will be 50% to 80% less and mid-cycle pains due to ovulation will usually be cured by the combined OCP. Mild cases of endometriosis can often be controlled by the combined OCP with beneficial effects upon future fertility.

4. The combined pill may help some women with pre-menstrual syndrome or pre-menopausal symptoms due to imbalances or deficiencies in their own sex hormones. This is because it supplies a steady amount of synthetic hormones which suppress or compensate for unpleasant hormonal highs and lows. Pre-menopausal women may find that their vaginal lubrication and sexual function is helped by the combined OCP and it certainly protects their bones against calcium loss. Once the menopause arrives, the OCP should be replaced with natural Hormone Replacement Therapy. Women over 45 who have not had a natural menstrual period for over twelve months can generally be considered menopausal although this should be confirmed with blood tests. Other favourable hormonal effects of the combined OCP may be an improvement in some types of inflammatory diseases such as rheumatoid arthritis and thyroid disease.

5. Many women will be delighted to know that a special "tailor-made" combined OCP can cure acne, pimples, oily hair and excessive facial and body hair. An ideal tailor-made pill for these problems consists of two separate hormones — oestrogen in the form of ethinyl oestradiol (Estigyn) 30 to 50mcg daily and cyproterone acetate (Androcur) 2.5mg to 5 mg daily. Both of these hormones are taken together for three weeks on and one week off.

Women in Europe, Australia and New Zealand are able to obtain a contraceptive pill called 'Diane' containing both Estigyn and Androcur combined in one pill and in these countries Diane is the most popular type of pill prescribed. Why not take an OCP that promotes feminine skin and hair if given the choice?

If you suffer with more severe degrees of acne or superfluous hair, higher doses of Androcur will be required, at least initially. (Refer to Chapter 8 for details).

6. In women anxious about the small size of their breasts, the OCP, particularly brands with a higher oestrogen content, often produces a desirable increase in breast size.

7. Many women with infrequent menstruation can benefit by taking the combined OCP. Generally speaking, women who often miss their periods for several months to six months at a time (a condition known as amenorrhoea) have a problem with the function of their ovaries. They may have too little oestrogen production from their ovaries (especially if they are underweight and sportive), or too much oestrogen and male hormone production from their ovaries (especially if they are overweight with skin problems). Those with too little oestrogen run an increased risk of osteoporosis and fractures of the spine and hips while those with too much oestrogen face an increased risk of uterine cancer. By correcting these hormonal imbalances, the combined OCP prevents osteoporosis and uterine cancer if taken regularly in women with infrequent menstruation. Of course, when they start the combined oral contraceptive pill their menstruation becomes regular.

The Combined OCP and The Risk of Cancer

If you are on the combined OCP you have less chance of developing cancer of the ovary and uterus and this protective effect lasts for approximately fifteen years after coming off the pill.

You will also have less chance of non-cancerous (benign) breast lumps. The effect of this pill upon your risk of breast cancer is not so clear and may vary depending upon the age at which you started the pill and for how long you took it.

The Harvard University study of over 120,000 nurses aged 30 to 55 published in the Journal of the National Cancer Institute found no link between the use of the combined OCP and breast cancer, even in cases where this pill was taken for an extended time. Studies of women aged less than 45 who had used the pill before the age of 25 have shown an increasing relative risk of breast cancer with years of pill use, especially in women who have never given birth. (See Reference 2). Two European studies have found an increased risk of breast cancer in women who started the pill at an early age, but the United States Federal Drug Administration believes that existing evidence does not support a change in prescription and use of the combined OCP.

More research is needed to determine the risk of breast cancer associated with combined OCP use at a young age because women who have taken the pill when young are only now reaching the age where the breast cancer risk is highest. This research should also examine the interaction of the pill with diet, exercise and lifestyle factors in determining its long term effects upon cancer.

Young women should be told that there may be a slightly increased risk of breast cancer from long-term use of the combined OCP, if they are to give valid informed consent when making choices in their method of contraception.

The effect of the combined OCP upon cancer of the cervix also needs more research as one study has shown an increased incidence in women on the OCP, especially after ten years' use, but cause and effect has not been proven. (See Reference 3). Thus, it is most important that all women on the OCP have regular annual pap smears.

Side Effects of the Combined OCP

When the OCP was first introduced thirty years ago, its high doses of synthetic hormones were far more likely to induce side effects such as nausea, headaches, weight gain, high blood pressure, blood clots, heart attacks and strokes, than today's low dose OCPs. Indeed, the original OCP was more suited to an elephant than a woman! We are still searching for the ideal contraceptive and although today's low-dose OCPs are generally safe and well tolerated, they are not without side effects in all women. Let's explore some possible side effects:

1. Weight Gain

Some women are definitely susceptible to this, particularly those who are always battling with their weight. OCPs containing the more masculine (androgenic) progestogens, particularly in higher dose pills, may stimulate the appetite and increase the accumulation of body fat. Pills containing a high dose of oestrogen may cause fluid retention which further increases weight. This fluid retention may be associated with an aggravation of varicose veins, leg cramps or aching legs.

2. Nausea and/or Vomiting

This is similar to the "morning sickness" of pregnancy and is due to the effect of the pill's hormones upon the liver and stomach. Thankfully, it is often temporary. If you have gall bladder disease or gall stones, the OCP often aggravates these problems causing nausea and abdominal pains. The risk of liver tumours (which are very rare) is slightly increased in women who take high dose OCPs for a prolonged period.

3. Breakthrough Bleeding

This is defined as bleeding while you are taking the OCP and occurs apart from your regular withdrawal bleed. Because it is usually unpredictable, it is a real nuisance but may be prevented by changing to a higher dose pill. It may be a signal that your OCP is not being properly absorbed from your intestines which may occur if you have an intestinal upset or infection or if you are on other medication (e.g. antibiotics, anti-epileptic drugs, or asthma medication). Please check with your doctor if it is occurring as adequate contraception may not be ensured.

4. Pigmentation of the Skin

The OCP and also pregnancy may induce brown patches of pigmentation, especially on the face, and this is called chloasma or the "mask of pregnancy".

5. Absence of Menstruation (Amenorrhoea)

One in every hundred women on the combined OCP fails to menstruate after stopping the pill. Such women usually have pre-existing hormonal problems such as the polycystic ovarian syndrome (See Page 97) and their menstrual cycle can be restored with hormonal therapy thus restoring their fertility. The OCP does not exert any long-term negative effects on fertility.

6. Mood Changes

The effect of the OCP upon a woman's mental and emotional state is variable. Some find that it increases wellbeing and equanimity by preventing hormonal highs and lows, whereas others find it induces depression, irritability and loss of sexual desire. The latter effect probably arises because the pill reduces the amount of the brain chemical serotonin that exerts a balancing effect upon moods, mental drive, appetite and sexual desire. In a minority of women, the OCP induces severe and unpleasant mood changes that necessitate its discontinuation. Thankfully, the mood disorders go quickly after stopping the OCP.

7. Headaches

Headaches, especially of the migrainous type may be aggravated or brought on for the first time by the combined OCP. If severe migraine occurs, especially if associated with visual or neurological disturbance (e.g. blindness, flashing lights, weakness or numbness of body parts, speech disturbance, etc), the OCP must be stopped immediately.

8. Disorders of the Circulation

The high dose OCPs of the 1960s and early 70s were associated with an increased risk of cardiovascular disorders such as high blood pressure, blood clots, heart attacks and strokes. These risks have been greatly reduced with the use of much lower doses of synthetic hormones in today's modern OCPs and are mainly confined to women over 35 who smoke or have pre-existing cardiovascular risk factors, such as high blood pressure, hardening of the arteries or diabetes.

Modern low dose combined OCPs can be considered safe, but only in "safe women", as they can be dangerous in "dangerous women". Dangerous women are smokers, diabetics, those with high blood pressure, obesity, blood clots, high cholesterol or a previous or family history of heart attacks, angina and strokes.

Smoking is a far greater risk factor for heart disease than the combined OCP. Women over the age of 35 who are on the combined OCP and smoke should either give up the pill or stop smoking. I believe that any woman who smokes regardless of her age, should not take the combined OCP because of the combined harmful effects of the OCP and smoking upon the blood vessels.

Safe women are those who do not have any of the risk factors characterising dangerous women and according to the Fertility and Maternal Health Drugs Advisory Committee of the Federal Drug Administration, safe women may continue to take a low dose combined OCP up to any age and, if desired, up until the menopause. Even so, safe women over the age of 40.who take the combined OCP may slightly increase their risk of cardiovascular disease and if this is found unacceptable, the mini pill (POP) is a good alternative.

The synthetic hormones in the pill tend to increase the blood fats, cholesterol and triglycerides, but these increases are usually slight and not outside of normal limits. You can have your blood fats measured before starting and again after six months of taking the OCP to detect any adverse changes.

Ideally, all women should have their blood pressure checked two to three months after starting the OCP to make sure that any increase is not excessive.

Women on the combined OCP who have major surgery are much more likely to get post-operative blood clots. So if you are scheduled for planned surgery you should be taken off the combined OCP four to six weeks prior to the surgery. Emergency surgery should be preceded by drug therapy to prevent blood clots.

Overall, if you have any cardiovascular risk factors, the combined OCP acts to multiply them. The lower the dose of hormones in the OCP, the safer it is and you should work with your doctor to find the lowest dose OCP that works for you.

Women Who Should Not Take The Combined OCP

There are certain conditions that preclude you from taking the combined OCP:

1. Oestrogen-sensitive cancers such as uterine or breast cancer. The cause of unexplained vaginal bleeding should be diagnosed before beginning any OCP;

2. Active liver disease or liver tumours;

3. Severe or frequent migraine headaches;

4. Some medical conditions such as porphyria or diabetes;

5. Cardiovascular diseases such as blood clots, heart disease, strokes, high blood pressure, very high cholesterol and triglycerides.

Contraception in the Future

No one has yet found the ideal hormone contraceptive although we are getting close.

In particular, experts agree that it is best to use the smallest dose of synthetic hormones and also to use a progesterone that is "friendly" to our blood fats and cardiovascular system. These friendly progesterones are non-masculine (non-androgenic) and are also friendly to our skin as they are more feminine and help to control acne and facial hair. Examples of these friendly feminine progesterones are cyproterone acetate, desogestrel and gestodene.

In Europe, Australia and New Zealand, women have access to OCPs containing smaller doses (20 mcg as opposed to 30 mcg) of oestrogen combined with friendly progesterones such as desogestrel. Brand names of these pills are Mercilon, Marvelon and Diane and these are ideal OCPs for older women or indeed for the majority of women.

TABLE 4: OCP SIDE EFFECTS

SIDE EFFECT	AVOID	USE	OTHER MEASURES
Weight gain	High dose pills	Mini pill (POP) Triphasic pills	Regular exercise Low-fat diet
Nausea, Vomiting	High dose pills	Mini pill (POP) Triphasic pills may be tolerated Progesterone hormone implant	Take OCP with food and vitamin B6
Breakthrough bleeding	Mini pill (POP) Low-dose pills	Higher dose pills or tailor-made OCP from your doctor	Take the OCP at the same time each day. See your doctor for a gynaecological examination
Facial pigmentation (Chloasma)	Combined OCPs	Mini pill (POP)	Sunscreen lotion Broad brim hat Depigmentation cream at night
Breast tenderness	High dose OCPs	Mini pill (POP) Triphasic OCPs Tailor-made OCP	Evening Primrose Oil 3000mg daily Femme Phase 2 tsps daily. Antioxidants
Mood disorders Poor libido	High dose OCPs Avoid masculine progesterones	Mini pill (POP) Tailor-made OCP	Zinc chelate 50 mg daily Femme Phase 2 tsps daily Magnesium 500 mg daily
Headaches, Migraines	All combined OCPs	Mini pill (POP)	Increase water intake. Evening Primrose Oil 3000 mg daily Magnesium 500 to 1000 mg daily Vitamin E 500 iu
High Blood Pressure Blood Clots	All combined OCPs	Mini pill (POP) Progesterone hormone implant	Vitamin C, garlic Fish oil 1000 mg daily 2 litres water daily
Vaginal Candida	High dose OCPs	Triphasic OCPs or mini pill	Low sugar diet, garlic Antioxidants Acidophilus

Hormone Implants

These contain the synthetic progesterone levonorgestrel and are inserted under the skin into the fat. They release a small amount of hormone every day which is only one quarter to one half of that obtained from current OCPs and so are very safe. They are very reliable contraceptives with a failure rate around one-tenth that of the OCP.

The most outstanding thing about the implant is that it provides continuous contraception for five years! Because hormone implants at this stage contain potent androgenic progesterones they may induce side effects such as weight gain and headaches and by the time we have them in Australia, researchers may have developed an implant with a more natural or feminine progesterone.

Hormone Patches

These adhesive patches are impregnated with synthetic hormones that are slowly absorbed into the blood stream through the skin and provide constant low dose contraception. The patches could be applied to the skin of the upper inside thigh and changed every third day. They will be safer than oral forms of contraception and their arrival is eagerly awaited.

Vaginal Rings

The vaginal ring is a flexible silicone rubber ring, similar in size to a vaginal diaphragm (See Diagram 10) and is impregnated with synthetic hormones. It is placed high up in the vagina around the cervix where it slowly releases its hormones that are absorbed into the circulation thereby preventing ovulation.

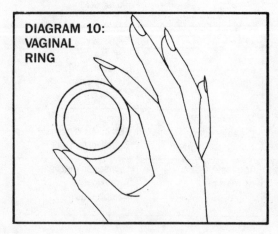

DIAGRAM 10: VAGINAL RING

Rings containing both oestrogen and progesterone are left inside the vagina for three weeks and then removed for one week to allow a menstrual bleed to occur. The ring is then reinserted by the woman to begin another monthly cycle. Rings containing only progesterone can be left in place for ninety days, before a new ring is needed.

Women generally find the vaginal rings easy and simple to use.

In trials the vaginal ring is proving to be very safe as it provides constant low doses of hormones and does not affect the metabolism of the liver to the same degree as hormone tablets. The vaginal ring is still on trial overseas. In Australia, the Sydney Centre for Research into Reproductive Health intends to start trials on its efficiency and it should be available here within several years.

The contraceptive hormone implant, vaginal ring and patch will be more effective than the mini pill because there is no risk of forgetting a daily pill.

References

1. Washington A.E, Gob S, Schachter J et al., *Chlamydia and PID: a word of caution about protection.* JAMA 1985; 253:2246-2250.

2. Schlesselman JJ., *Cancer of the Breast in relation to OCPs.* Contraception 1989; 40(1):1-38.

3. Beral V, et al, Results from the Royal College of GP's OCP study, Lancet 1988; 2:131-134.

CHAPTER 7

SURGICAL STERILIZATION
MAY BE MORE THAN YOU BARGAINED FOR

Surgical sterilization in a woman is known as tubal ligation and is a surgical procedure that interrupts or blocks the fallopian tube of the uterus. This prevents the egg from meeting with the sperm so that fertilization which normally occurs inside the fallopian tube cannot occur (See Diagram 11).

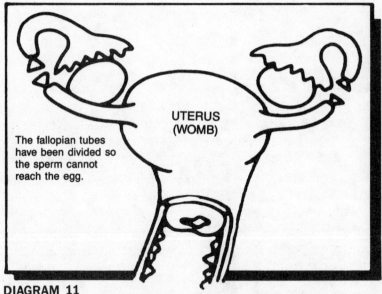

UTERUS (WOMB)

The fallopian tubes have been divided so the sperm cannot reach the egg.

DIAGRAM 11

It is a permanent form of sterilization and no one should undergo it unless they are absolutely certain that they do not want any more children. Surgical reversal of a tubal ligation can be attempted, but it does not always succeed. Micro surgical reversal of tubal ligation can give pregnancy rates as high as 70%, but a 100% guarantee can never be given and so at the outset it should be considered irreversible. Even if the fallopian tubes can be rejoined with micro surgery it is often impossible to rejoin the ovarian blood vessels that may have been divided or damaged at tubal ligation. Pregnancy following reversal of tubal ligation may be associated with hormonal imbalances, miscarriage or poor growth of the baby and may require hormonal therapy.

Tubal ligation is a very commonly performed operation — with approximately 650,000 American and 50,000 Australian women undergoing it every year.

It is often taken very casually with many women believing it is the easiest thing to do, once their family is complete. Indeed, having your "tubes tied" seems so simple — no more pills or messy diaphragms to remember, just one day in hospital and you're on your way free of the worry of pregnancy. There is no doubt that tubal ligation is effective contraception as the failure rate is very low with three pregnancies in every 1,000 sterilized women. However, it is not always hassle-free and without side effects as you will soon see, and it is a pity that women undergoing or considering tubal ligation as a method of contraception are not always advised of all its possible long-term effects.

Techniques of Tubal Ligation

The fallopian tubes may be obstructed by different methods such as cutting, tying (Pomeroy technique), burning with an electric current or clipping them with metal or plastic rings or clips.

It is important that you check which method your surgeon will use as each method has different risks and complications associated with it.

1. The technique of **burning the tubes** (tubal diathermy) is now outmoded and should not be done as it is associated with a high chance of causing damage to the surrounding blood vessels, organs and intestines and the formation of scar tissue. It has a higher failure rate than clipping the tubes and is more likely to cause heavy menstrual periods in the future.

2. **Cutting or tying the tubes** (Pomeroy technique) has been used for many years and is the method used if sterilization is done immediately after childbirth. It has several disadvantages — an abdominal incision or laparotomy is required, it has a higher failure rate than clipping the tubes, the area of damage to the tubes and surrounding blood vessels is higher than clipping with more chance of damaging the blood supply to the ovary. If it is performed immediately after childbirth, it is a tragedy if anything goes wrong with the baby and it subsequently dies as the Pomeroy technique is not easily reversed.

3. If you are absolutely sure that you want a tubal ligation, the best method to ask for is **clipping of the tubes** which can be done through a laparoscope (long narrow telescope) that is inserted into the abdominal cavity through a half-inch incision. The laparoscope uses fiberoptics and functions like a hollow flash light so that the surgeon can see your organs and insert surgical tools through the hollow bore of the laparoscope. The tubes are compressed with a silastic ring (Falope ring) or metal clips (Filschie clips). The falope ring acts like a rubber band on the tubes and the filschie clips act like a metal staple and clamp the tubes closed. **In the hands of a good and experienced surgeon clipping of the tubes is less likely to cause damage to the surrounding blood vessels that supply the ovary and should be less likely to result in long-term problems with the function of the ovaries.** Clipping the tubes causes damage to a much smaller area of the tubes than either the burning or tying techniques and so is more easily reversed if you should change your mind. The falope rings and filschie clips are the safest technique with less risk of complications post-operatively.

Post-operative problems after tubal ligation such as haemorrhage, bowel damage, infections, peritonitis, blood clots, damage to surrounding organs and severe post-operative pain occur in 3% to 5% of cases. However, surgeons experienced in the technique of clipping the tubes tell me that this method has less than a 1% chance of such complications.

The technique of plugging or sealing the tubes at the points where they open into the uterus can be done through a hysteroscope, i.e. a telescope

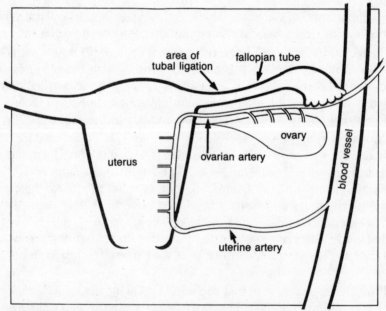

DIAGRAM 12: BLOOD SUPPLY TO OVARY AND UTERUS

84

passed into the uterine cavity through the cervix. This technique avoids any incisions being made but it is rarely reversible and has not as yet been perfected in the hands of many surgeons.

Currently, with all available methods of tubal ligation, there exists a chance (which varies between methods used) of damaging the blood supply to the ovary as the ovarian blood vessels run alongside the fallopian tubes on their way to the ovary (See Diagram 12). It is easy to see how these blood vessels could be compressed or cut during surgery to the closely adjacent tube.

Researchers in Australia have shown that the effects of blocking the blood supply to the ovarian artery is high blood pressure in the ovary which could result in the tissues of the ovary being damaged. If this occurs, the ovary may not function normally and its production of the sex hormones oestrogen and progesterone which depends upon adequate blood and oxygen supply may be reduced. In the future, more precise microsurgical techniques of tubal ligation, with careful conservation of the ovaries blood supply would provide a less hit and miss approach to the chances of long-term problems with ovarian function.

What Are The Possible Problems After a Tubal Ligation?

1. Menstrual and gynaecological problems

Since 1951, there have been reports in the literature that women have a higher risk of heavy menstrual bleeding, irregular bleeding and hysterectomy after tubal ligation. The incidence of pelvic pain, period pains, longer periods and pain during sexual intercourse may also be higher. Endometriosis may also be more likely after surgical sterilization. These problems often get worse with increasing time after the tubal ligation. Another irony of tubal ligation is that it may increase your chances of needing a hysterectomy in the future, although many women believe that it will provide an end to their contraceptive and gynaecological problems. (See Page 94 for References 1 to 6).

A study in the U.S. in 1951, followed up 200 women after tubal ligation. At least 16.5% of these women developed abnormal bleeding requiring a hysterectomy within ten years of sterilization which was three times more than the hysterectomy rate in non-sterilized women. A Scottish study found that the hysterectomy rate after tubal ligation was 9.3% compared to 2.5% in non-sterilized women.

Many surgeons minimise these complications refusing to admit that they have any relationship with tubal ligation and ascribe them to the fact that the patient is getting older, has come off the oral contraceptive pill since sterilization, and would have developed these problems anyway. Therefore, it is difficult to gauge the true incidence of subsequent gynaecological problems linked to tubal ligation.

If tubal ligation fails and pregnancy occurs, then there is a greater possibility of this being a tubal or ectopic pregnancy.

2. Hormonal problems

Some researchers believe that hormonal deficiencies and imbalances may affect up to 90% of women after tubal ligation and this area urgently needs more scientific scrutiny. Some women do escape any significant hormonal problems after tubal ligation, while others experience symptoms due to oestrogen deficiency or imbalances of oestrogen and progesterone.

The chances of hormonal problems depend upon damage to the ovarian blood supply and is higher if burning or tying/cutting techniques were used in the tubal ligation. The production of oestrogen from the ovary is more likely to be affected than is the production of progesterone, as oestrogen needs more oxygen for the many steps necessary in its synthesis by the ovary. If the ovarian blood supply is reduced by tubal ligation, the supply of oxygen to the ovary is diminished, resulting in inadequate oestrogen synthesis.

Women with inadequate amounts of oestrogen in their body will typically complain of loss of libido, fatigue, loss of feminine physique, difficulty in losing weight, vaginal dryness, bladder problems, reduced orgasms, poor memory and musculoskeletal aches and pains. Because oestrogen is necessary for the maintenance of collagen, women with low oestrogen levels after tubal ligation often complain of more rapid ageing of the skin and aches and pains as collagen is lost from the skin and bones. (Refer to the Oestrogen Level Score Chart on page 87 to see if you are lacking oestrogen).

The long-term effects of inadequate oestrogen production from the ovary, especially in younger women undergoing tubal ligation, are very harmful and increase the risk of cardiovascular disease and osteoporosis.

Women lacking both oestrogen and progesterone usually complain of mood disorders, fatigue, pre-menstrual syndrome and menstrual disturbances. Understandably, women with these hormonal problems are at greater risk of marital and family discord.

The development of such hormonal problems can be gradual and insidious, especially if not recognised for what they are, and may take several years after tubal ligation to fully develop. I have seen many women with such problems who were searching for an answer.

The symptoms that are characteristic of oestrogen deficiency may be grouped together in a chart and scored according to the following scale:

Absent = 0   Mild = 1   Moderate = 2   Severe = 3

TABLE 5: OESTROGEN LEVEL SCORE CHART

OESTROGEN DEFICIENCY SYMPTOM	SCORE (0-3)
Depression and mood changes	
Anxiety and/or irritability	
Unloved or unwanted feelings	
Poor memory and concentration	
Poor sleeping patterns (insomnia)	
Fatigue	
Backache	
Joint pains, increase in arthritis	
Muscle pains	
New facial hair	
Dry skin and/or sudden wrinkling	
Crawling, itching, burning sensations in the skin	
Reduced sexual desire	
Frequency or burning of urination	
Discomfort during sexual intercourse	
Vaginal dryness	
Hot flushes and/or excessive sweating	
Light-headedness or dizziness	
Headaches	
YOUR TOTAL SCORE:	

This chart is derived from Professor Nordin's Menopause Questionnaire, Institute of Medical & Veterinary Science, Adelaide, South Australia.

If your total score for all of these symptoms is 15 or more, then it is likely that you are suffering with a deficiency of oestrogen. If your score is around 30, your body is crying out for oestrogen. This can be confirmed or refuted with a simple blood test to check your level of oestrogen and Follicle Stimulating Hormone.

It is an interesting exercise to score your symptoms of oestrogen deficiency before and after commencing Hormone Replacement Therapy.

DON'T LET YOUR HORMONES RUIN YOUR LIFE

The Story of Virginia

Virginia was a prolific writer of children's stories and was finding it more and more difficult to use her word processor because of pain in her neck, forearms and wrists. The shopping and picking up her two young children were also proving stressful as she had lower back pain which restricted her bending over. She felt rather cheated and angry by these symptoms as she was only 39 and was suffering with symptoms that both she and her doctor thought were typical of a woman much older. She was not used to this as she had previously been very sportive and fit.

It had all started three years after her tubal ligation which had been performed immediately after the caesarean section required for the birth of her last child. She became increasingly exhausted which was due to undiagnosed anaemia due to her heavy painful periods that had developed in the last six months. Her beautiful athletic physique had also changed and she had developed lumpy cellulite around her buttocks and thighs although she was following a very healthy low fat diet. She found that her skin looked thinner and dry and started to age more rapidly.

Virginia's creativity also seemed to be flagging and the magical stories did not flow from her brain with the same ease and colour. She could not understand why she felt so down as she was trying to do all the right things and even her supplements of evening primrose oil, vitamins and minerals did not give her a lift.

Fortunately, Virginia's doctor had the foresight to refer her to a specialist as he remembered how different she had been four years ago and he suspected she had a hormonal problem. The specialist ordered blood and urine tests and discovered that Virginia had subnormal levels of oestrogen and progesterone, as well as a severe iron deficiency anaemia. She was started on iron supplements, given an oestrogen implant and natural oestrogen tablets to take along with progesterone. The progesterone tablets were to be taken for twelve days of every calendar month.

Within six weeks Virginia felt her aches and pains disappear and her mental and emotional state improved. Once again, she was churning out her children's stories and felt like playing with her children. She was delighted to find the lumpy cellulite reducing without having to starve herself to death and she now had the energy to resume her aerobics classes at the gym.

Virginia still felt a little cheated as her gynaecologist had not warned her that tubal ligation can result in hormonal problems and she felt that she was rather young to start Hormone Replacement Therapy. Had she known, she would never have had her tubes tied.

At least her symptoms had been recognised for what they were, or else she feared that she may have continued to age rapidly and needed anti-inflammatory drugs. Virginia was amazed that the hormone oestrogen exerted such a powerful influence in her body as she had never before been a victim of her hormones.

Can Hormone Problems After Tubal Ligation Be Treated?

In many women with hormonal problems after tubal ligation, a hormonal state similar to the pre-menopause is found. This means that the hormonal output from the ovaries is reduced to a similar level that we find typically in a woman in her late 40s who is approaching the menopause.

To assess the level of oestrogen and progesterone production by your ovaries you can ask your doctor to measure the amount of these hormones and their metabolites (breakdown products) in both blood and urine tests. If your doctor does not want to do this, ask for a referral to a specialist who is called a gynaecological endocrinologist. You have a right to know as it is vitally important because long-term consequences of oestrogen and progesterone deficiency could be an increased risk of cardiovascular disease, osteoporosis, premature ageing or cancer.

Oestrogen and progesterone production is best assessed in 24-hour urine tests the day before, during and after ovulation. Blood tests for levels of oestrogen, progesterone and Follicle Stimulating Hormone are also helpful, but because the daily production of oestrogen from the ovary fluctuates markedly, this may make one or two blood samples unreliable as true indications of your overall oestrogen state. This is best assessed in three separate 24-hour urine collections which integrate these fluctuations.

Once your doctor has proven that you have a hormonal deficiency or imbalance, this can be treated with natural Hormone Replacement Therapy.

It is possible to supplement your own inadequate oestrogen levels with natural oestrogen in the form of tablets which can be taken every day. Make sure your doctor uses the natural form of oestrogen as synthetic forms do not work.

Some women will also need oestrogen replacement in the form of an **oestrogen implant**. The implants consist of small pellets of pure crystalline oestradiol and resemble a tiny piece of spaghetti. They come in various strengths to suit individual needs and are somewhat expensive, although the cost can be claimed from some private health funds. They can be painlessly implanted into the fatty layer of your abdomen or buttocks under a local anaesthetic and many doctors use a small hollow tube with a sharp cutting edge to slide the pellet neatly into your fat. (See Diagram 13.)

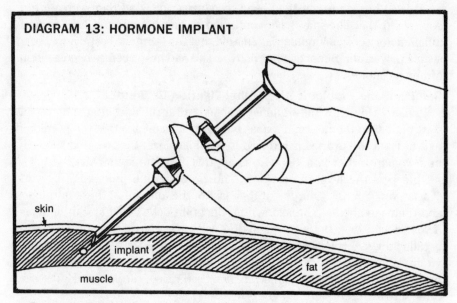

DIAGRAM 13: HORMONE IMPLANT

skin

implant

fat

muscle

Depending upon the strength of the implant chosen by your doctor, an implant will continue to release oestrogen directly into your blood stream for between four to twelve months which is ideal for those who cannot remember to take tablets.

Of all the types of HRT, an implant comes closest to copying the function of your own ovaries as in both cases oestrogen is released directly into the bloodstream and carried to the various oestrogen-dependent tissues of your body. Thus, your hungry cells get their supply of precious oestrogen before the liver enzymes can break it down. Unfortunately, this is not so with oestrogen tablets which are first broken down by passage through the liver after their absorption from the gut. Thus, the liver could be said to weaken the effect of oestrogen tablets upon your cells, whereas the oestrogen implant is able to deliver an unweakened supply of oestrogen.

Oestrogen can be given via your vagina and indeed this is a very popular form of HRT. It is easily inserted with a vaginal applicator which enables you to place the cream high into the vagina. It is best done last thing at night on retiring, after sex, and after emptying your bladder. Oestrogen will be rapidly absorbed through the vaginal lining into the bloodstream and reasonable levels of blood oestrogens can be achieved.

Oestrogen replacement can also be given in the form of an **oestrogen patch** which is a sticky transparent membrane impregnated with natural oestrogen. It is applied to the skin of the buttock, abdomen or trunk (excluding the breast) and releases oestrogen to the skin which absorbs it into your bloodstream. The patch is changed every third day.

Thus, oestrogen replacement is very versatile and different combinations of the oestrogen tablets, patches, implants and creams can be tried with your own doctor until you find the programme that suits your individual mental, physical and sexual requirements.

No matter what type of oestrogen replacement you receive, it is necessary that you also receive replacement with the other ovarian hormone progesterone. This is usually given in tablet form and must be given for twelve to fourteen days of every calendar month to balance the oestrogen and regulate your cycle to bring on a regular menstrual bleed.

If your periods are very heavy and/or painful you may need to take both progesterone tablets and oestrogen tablets for twenty-five days of every calendar month, which is a similar programme to the oral contraceptive pill. However, the oral contraceptive pill should not be used routinely to treat women with hormonal problems after tubal ligation, as contraception is no longer required and it contains synthetic hormones which do not have the same beneficial effect in your body as natural oestrogen.

The Story of Ruth

Some women can also benefit from injections of natural hormones usually on a temporary basis. Ruth was an example of this type of treatment.

Ruth looked tired and depressed as she slumped into the chair on the other side of my desk. The most obvious reason for her fatigue was probably that she had five children all under ten years of age. However, as she related the sequence of her symptoms, the jigsaw pieces started coming together.

Two and a half years ago, Ruth had undergone surgical sterilization from a surgeon who had used the outmoded technique of burning the tubes. She had not been told what technique the surgeon would use as the consent form she had signed did not explore the alternatives. Ruth had thought this was her only way out as she could not tolerate the oral contraceptive pill and her husband refused vasectomy.

Eighteen months after her sterilisation she developed heavy painful periods heralded by increasing pre-menstrual tension with severe mood changes. She felt resentful towards her husband who could not understand her unpredictable moods and loss of interest in sex. She experienced a constant dull throbbing pain in her pelvis and sexual intercourse was acutely painful on deep penetration.

Ruth was nearly 40 and felt that her hormonal problems may be due to an early menopause, especially as she felt she was ageing rapidly. Her rapidly diminishing self esteem and confidence were not helped by her husband who felt that her symptoms were psychosomatic.

I asked her if she ever felt good. She replied that at the end of seven days of menstrual bleeding she felt a bit like her old self and said, "That's when I wear high heels again, cook cakes and take the kids out, but I only feel normal for seven days, then the rotten pre-menstrual syndrome takes the wind out of my sails".

Ruth wanted to know if she could have her tubal ligation reversed. I said this was doubtful as her surgeon had used the burning method which often causes damage to the fragile tubes and the blood supply to the ovaries. Trying to reverse this damage would be no guarantee to cure her hormonal problems and would also involve more surgery and pain.

I encouraged Ruth to try hormonal therapy. Blood and urine tests revealed that Ruth's ovaries were not functioning well presumably because of damage to their blood supply induced by burning of the tubes and blood vessels at the time of sterilization.

Ruth started on natural oestrogen tablets (Progynova 1mg twice daily) everyday and progesterone (Provera 5mg) for the first twelve days of every calendar month. The Provera tablets were necessary to balance the oestrogen and regulate her cycle and they would bring on a menstrual period around the twelfth day of every calendar month.

This treatment relieved her pre-menstrual tension, depression, pelvic pain and heavy bleeding and she started to get on top of things again.

Her flagging libido remained a problem and so we checked her level of male hormones which are necessary for a healthy sex drive, orgasmic ability and so called "feminine virility". We found that her male hormones were almost non-existent which explained why she felt asexual which she described as "almost like a eunuch".

Ruth and I decided that this was best overcome by giving her an injection of natural oestrogen and testosterone (Primodian Depot injection) every three months, with this injection being given at the end of every third menstrual period. This was to continue for nine to twelve months and would build up her body's male hormones to a degree sufficient to increase libido but without causing side effects such as facial hair or acne. The Primodian injection proved nothing short of miraculous and Ruth began to feel like a vital, sexual and happy human being for the first time in three years.

There are thousands of women like Ruth who are standing on the sidelines, struggling with their health and waiting for enlightened doctors to draw the curtains on the astounding benefits of natural hormone replacement.

Until more long-term studies of women after tubal ligation are available, we can only guess at the number of women having hysterectomies to relieve their post-sterilization symptoms. They should be given all the alternatives to hysterectomy and not be told that it is the only answer.

Precautions Before Having A Tubal Ligation

As has been seen, surgical sterilization or tubal ligation is not always free of hassles and should not be taken casually. I would not advise my patients to undergo tubal ligation unless a further pregnancy would be a catastrophe as in women with severe diabetes, heart, kidney or liver disease. I believe that with current non-surgical methods of contraception and the newer oral contraceptive pills, vaginal rings and contraceptive implants that are imminent, that the benefits of tubal ligation do not outweigh the risks. I would advise any woman with gynaecological problems such as heavy, painful bleeding, fibroids, endometriosis, pelvic pain, pre-menstrual syndrome or a past history of nasty, postnatal depression to avoid tubal ligation.

Until surgeons have perfected and standardised surgical techniques (preferably microsurgical) for tubal ligation, I think that younger women considering this operation should seriously think about the possibility that current techniques (which vary widely) may put them at risk for years of hormonal and gynaecological problems and reduced ovarian function.

Older women may have little to gain from tubal ligation. They already face the likelihood of diminished ovarian function in the pre-menopausal years and tubal ligation will give them less contraceptive time than younger women. Furthermore, they are less fertile anyway so that simple and safe contraceptive methods such as the progesterone only pill, diaphragms and vaginal rings and hormone implants are relatively more effective.

If you really want a tubal ligation, make sure that your personal life is stable and happy. I have seen many women who later wanted a reversal of their tubal ligation. If you are currently taking the oral contraceptive pill and are considering having a tubal ligation, come off the pill for six months before having the operation. If during this six-month break your periods are heavy or painful you are not a good candidate for a tubal ligation as this operation may increase these menstrual problems.

Before having a tubal ligation, have a thorough gynaecological examination, pelvic examination and pap smear and if you have abnormal bleeding, you should have a dilatation and curettage of the uterus. This will exclude the presence of cancer of the uterus or cervix or huge fibroids, that may require a hysterectomy in the near future, in which case a tubal ligation would have been an entirely unnecessary and unpleasant experience.

Finally, I believe that the consent forms for tubal ligation should be expanded to include all the potential complications and problems (including the increased risk of hysterectomy) that may occur in the long term subsequent to this procedure. The consent form should also state that more research is needed to determine the real incidence of these problems. Then we could say that women are really able to give valid informed consent to a surgical procedure that may have a lasting effect upon their lives.

References

Many scientific studies expose the reality of post-tubal ligation disorders and confirm that pre-existing menstrual problems can be worsened by sterilization.

1. De Stefano, et al, *Long term risk of menstrual disturbance after tubal sterilization,* Am.J.Obstet. and Gynaecol., Aug.1, 1985, Vol 152. No.7 pt.1, pp 835-841.

2. *Factors seen as links to post-tubal ligation syndrome* Contraception Tech. Update, Feb 1986, Vol. 7, No. 2, pp. 13-15.

3. Cattanach J., *Oestrogen deficiency after tubal ligation*, Lancet, April 13, 1985, 1(8433) pp. 847-849.

4. Stock, R.J., *Sequelae of tubal ligation: An analysis of 75 consecutive hysterectomies* South. Med. J., Oct. 1984, Vol. 77, No. 10, pp 1255-1260.

5. Cattanach J., *Post-tubal sterilization problems correlated with ovarian steroidogenesis,* Contraception, Nov 1988, Vol. 38, No. 5.

6. Templeton AA, *Hysterectomy following sterilization*, British Journal Obstetrics & Gynaecology; Oct 1982, Vol. 89, No. 10, pp 845-888.

CHAPTER 8

HOW YOUR HORMONES AFFECT YOUR APPEARANCE

When the body's hormones do not balance, dramatic and devastating changes in physical appearance and demeanour can take place. Let us look at the most influential of these imbalances.

TOO MANY MALE HORMONES

Male hormones in women are normal, provided that less of them are produced than in men. There are several male hormones, the best known being testosterone but in reality these hormones are just as much female as male; the only difference being that women normally produce much less of them than men. Indeed, male hormones are essential to normal female wellbeing and increase sex drive, physical endurance, mental drive, self-assertiveness and improve mood and confidence. They can help us to cope with physical and mental stress and can be powerful anti-depressants in both sexes.

There are several specific male hormones, also known as androgens or anabolic steroids.

The female ovary secretes three main male hormones called testosterone, androstenedione and dehydroepiandrosterone. Male hormones are also produced by the adrenal glands, liver, fat and skin. In a woman's normal menstrual cycle the blood level of male hormones increases at mid-cycle about the time of ovulation, and this is why women are most sexy at this time.

For women it is most desirable that a correct balance of male hormones is maintained because if they become excessive, masculine changes can occur in the appearance. Let us take a look at how excessive amounts of male hormones can affect your body hair, scalp hair and skin.

Body Hair

Excessive male hormones can lead to an increase in hair on areas of the body where hair is normally prominent only in males. You would notice an increase in hair on your chin, upper lip, the side of your face, chest, lower abdomen and thighs. This problem is called **hirsutism** and it troubles about 20 to 30% of all women in varying degrees, which explains the high frequency of advertisements in women's magazines for centres removing excessive facial and body hair. Most women with hirsutism have only a mild degree and do not have any serious hormonal imbalances which would lead to irreversible masculinisation.

What Causes Hirsutism?

The hair follicles are sensitive to male hormones and increasing levels of these hormones promote the rate of hair growth and the transformation of fine, soft or "vellus" hair to coarser "terminal" hair. This effect occurs in hair on the face and the body but not on the scalp.

The most common cause of hirsutism is a slight over-production of male hormones from the ovaries and from the adrenal glands. This slight increase in ovarian and/or adrenal male hormones can be detected in blood tests and although it does not cause any ill-effects upon health or fertility, it does stimulate the annoying growth of body hair. In some women with mild hirsutism, blood levels of male hormones are completely normal and the fault lies in excessive sensitivity of their skin and hair follicles to normal levels of male hormones.

There is often a family history of hirsutism in related females and it occurs most commonly in women of Southern-European and Middle-Eastern descent. Racial and **genetic factors** are obviously important. Hirsutism is rare among oriental women.

Women who are **overweight** are more likely to suffer with hirsutism because their excessive amounts of fat are associated with higher levels of male hormones. If they lose weight, their levels of male hormones usually decrease with a corresponding reduction in body and facial hair.

The gynaecological disorder of **polycystic ovaries** can cause hirsutism. In this condition, the ovaries may become enlarged and develop many small follicle cysts around the periphery. (See Diagram 14). This problem is quite common, and around one in every six women probably has a tendency to polycystic ovaries. These polycystic ovaries secrete excessive amounts of male hormones which may result in hirsutism, acne and infrequent menstruation. Many women with polycystic ovaries are overweight and should try to lose their excessive weight which may in itself restore regular menstruation and normal levels of male hormones. Conversely, if such women gain weight their menstrual periods become less frequent and acne and excess hair increase. In some obese women, it seems that excessive amounts of male hormones from their fat somehow "virilize" their ovaries stimulating them to produce excessive male hormones and this can become a vicious circle. The tendency to polycystic ovaries is inherited and may be triggered by stress or weight gain.

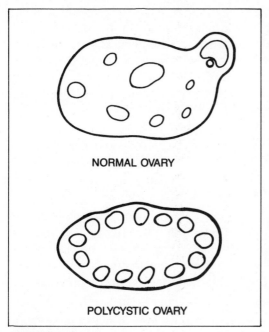

NORMAL OVARY

POLYCYSTIC OVARY

DIAGRAM 14

Some **medications** may increase body and facial hair such as the anabolic steroids used by athletes and body builders. Other drugs such as Danazol, Dilantin and some brands of the oral contraceptive pill containing the masculine progestogen norgestrel may also increase facial hair.

Hirsutism is generally mild to moderate in degree but if it is severe or of rapid onset and progression, tests must be done to check for a severe glandular disorder that may lead to extreme masculine changes in appearance called virilization.

Virilization

This describes the masculine changes that occur in women with very high levels of male hormones. In such cases there will be a dramatic and widespread increase in facial and body hair, greasy skin, acne, loss of menstruation and shrinkage of the breasts. It is usually frighteningly obvious as, in essence, a woman finds herself transforming into a man. She will notice recession of her scalp hairline with a male pattern of baldness, deepening of her voice, enlargement of her clitoris into a mini-penis and a defeminisation of her figure.

Virilization is a rare event and is always associated with a serious hormonal problem such as a tumour of the ovaries or adrenal glands. In such cases, these tumours produce large amounts of male hormones and blood tests reveal greatly increased levels of androgens that may be even greater than those found in males. These tumours may be malignant cancers and they may reveal themselves as obvious lumps or swellings in the pelvis or abdomen. They can be visualised on an ultrasound scan or cat scan of the pelvis and abdomen or by passing a telescope (laparoscope) through the abdominal wall.

Balding

Loss or thinning of the scalp hair is fairly common in women and usually causes a large amount of anxiety and stress. The medical term for loss of scalp hair is alopecia and if it is associated with increased levels of male hormones, it is called "androgenic alopecia". Alopecia is frequently associated with increased levels of male hormones. The most common underlying cause for this disorder is polycystic ovarian syndrome.

Androgenic alopecia may be of two types:

Male Pattern Androgenic Alopecia where the hair loss occurs in the areas of the temples and forehead producing a receding hairline. Women with this type of alopecia may have inherited this tendency from their father or grandfather.

Female Pattern Androgenic Alopecia where the hair loss is more diffuse or widespread. Hereditary factors are not important in this type of hair loss. Female Pattern Androgenic Alopecia may occur around the time of the menopause when the ovaries may increase their production of male hormones while their output of the female hormones is slowing down.

The effect of male hormones upon scalp hair is opposite to their effect upon facial and body hair. Whereas excessive male hormones increase facial and body hair, they reduce the growth of scalp hair. Excessive amounts or sensitivity to male hormones may interfere with the scalp hair growth cycle and cause a progressive loss of strong, thick-coloured "terminal" hair which is replaced only by fine, soft "vellus" hair which resembles baby hair. **The drug Androcur can be very helpful for balding women.**

The Story of Heather

Heather, a 59-year-old widow, had come to my surgery in a forlorn state. She had been consulting a dermatologist for several years to obtain treatment for hair loss from her scalp. When I examined her scalp there was a definite loss of hair as well as some circular areas on her scalp that had no hair at all. Heather had become anxious and had finally resorted to wearing a wig. She said that the steroid cortisone injections she was receiving into her scalp had been painful and ineffective.

Heather's hair loss had begun at the time of her natural menopause and she had also noticed an increase in unsightly facial hair at this time. Her blood sample revealed very low levels of oestrogen and elevated levels of testosterone (male hormone) which is a common finding in post-menopausal women not receiving Hormone Replacement Therapy. I explained to Heather that she had "Androgenic Alopecia" due to low levels of female hormones and excessive levels of male hormones (androgens).

I started Heather on a course of natural oestrogen and Androcur to reduce her level of male hormones. I also gave her nutritional supplements of Evening Primrose Oil, Zinc and Esten to ensure a glossy and healthy appearance to her skin and hair.

Nine months later, Heather's hair had improved dramatically although it was unfortunate that two of the circular patches that had been injected with steroids did not respond and remained bald. I concluded that in general it is best to avoid steroid injections into the scalp unless all other measures had failed. Nevertheless, Heather was pleased with the result and was able to conceal her small bald circles by cleverly rearranging her hair style. Heather was quite happy to continue the oestrogen and Androcur for many years, as they had stopped her facial hair and made her feel more feminine and attractive.

Acne

Male hormones stimulate the secretion of oily fluid from the skin's tiny glands which are called sebaceous glands. In susceptible women, this may result in acne of various types and degrees which begins at or soon after puberty and may persist well into the 20s and 30s and in some cases up to the menopause. Acne may be associated with a slightly raised level of male hormones from the ovaries or adrenal glands or may be due to an increased sensitivity of the skin's sebaceous glands to normal levels of male hormones. Women with polycystic ovaries often complain of moderate to severe acne along with their hirsutism.

PREVENTING THE PHYSICAL EFFECTS OF TOO MANY MALE HORMONES

Thankfully, it is now possible to prevent and reverse the masculine changes that result from excessive androgen production or activity. In years gone by, acne and facial hair have caused many women of all ages considerable stress and embarrassment in their social and professional lives. Uncontrolled acne in particular may lead to permanent scarring and disfigurement if allowed to continue but such women can now be promised near to perfect skin. I myself remember the extreme self-consciousness caused by my own adolescent acne and only wish that the doctor I had consulted way back then had known of the value of hormonal therapy in suppressing acne.

Overcoming Acne and Facial/Body Hair

For women with moderate to severe acne or facial hair, it is usually necessary to use drugs with a hormonal action that will either reduce the body's production of male hormones and/or block the action of male hormones upon the hair follicles and sebaceous glands in the skin. These drugs are extremely effective and, under strict medical supervision, are safe. They need to be given for a long time and you need to feel that the improvement in your appearance warrants the expense and slight risk in taking this long-term medication.

Because I am a naturopathic doctor as well as a medical doctor, I am often asked if nutritional supplements can cure acne, facial hair or thinning of scalp hair. Unfortunately, they will not cure these problems and although they may help, particularly with thinning of the scalp hair (See Table 6), hormonal therapy is the most effective strategy.

Let us take a look at some of the hormonal drugs that reduce the production and action of male hormones in our bodies.

Androcur

The chemical name for Androcur is cyproterone acetate and this remarkable drug acts like an anti-male hormone. **It is the most powerful anti-male hormone available providing an almost 100% cure of acne after three to nine months of use and reverses hirsutism in 80% of women after nine to twelve months of use.** Approximately one in every two women with androgenic alopecia (See Page 98) will obtain a regrowth or thickening of the scalp hair after using Androcur for nine to twelve months.

Androcur has been used overseas since 1974 and it is a component of the oral contraceptive pill called "Diane 35" which is commonly prescribed as a contraceptive in acne sufferers. Androcur is really a hormone with a dual action, being not only an anti-male hormone but also a progestogen and so it can be used with oestrogen in an oral contraceptive pill.

Androcur is given with the female hormone oestrogen on a cyclical basis in much the same way as the oral contraceptive pill is taken and this can be tailor-made for you to suppress acne and/or facial hair and to provide contraception. (See Table 6). This is important as women taking Androcur must avoid pregnancy because its anti-male hormone properties may stop the sexual development in a male foetus.

In post-menopausal women, or women who have had a hysterectomy, pregnancy is not a concern and so Androcur can be taken without regard to contraception.

Generally speaking, Androcur is well tolerated by most women and when it is given along with oestrogen, the side effects are similar to those of being on the oral contraceptive pill. (See Page 79).

Most women are overjoyed to have clear feminine skin which makes it easier to put up with any annoying side effects. Because Androcur is a potent anti-male hormone, high doses of it may cause a reduction in sex drive, reduced concentration, fatigue and mild depression.

TABLE 6: TREATMENT OF PROBLEMS
DUE TO EXCESSIVE MALE HORMONES

PROBLEMS	HORMONAL TREATMENT	OTHER DRUGS AND MEASURES
Acne	1. Estigyn (oestrogen) .03 to .05mg daily with Androcur 2.5 mg to 100mg for 2 or 3 weeks every month. 2. Aldactone 50 to 200mg daily or from day 5-26 of the menstrual cycle. 3. Oral contraceptive pill (OCP) by itself or with Androcur 2.5mg to 25mg daily or with Aldactone.	1. "Roaccutane" tablets are extremely effective for cystic acne but because they can cause birth defects they are only prescribed by skin specialists. 2. "Retin A" cream or lotion — is also anti-ageing. 3. Long-term antibiotics (may cause candida). 4. Antibiotic lotion e.g. Neomedrol. 5. Antioxidant 1 or 2 tablets daily
Excess Facial and Body Hair Hirsutism	4. Androcur 2.5mg to 100mg daily by itself or with a natural oestrogen in menopausal women or women after hysterectomy.	Under the supervision of a beautician: Plucking — not recommended Waxing — not for very coarse thick hair Bleaching — for moustache Depilatory creams Shaving — does not increase hair re-growth Electrolysis — for small areas only
Balding (Androgenic Alopecia)	5. Cortisone type drug e.g. dexamethasone 0.25mg to 0.5mg at night.	Check function of thyroid gland. Specific nutritional supplements may be very helpful such as: 1. Femme Phase, 2 tsps daily 2. Evening Primrose Oil 3000 mg daily 3. Zinc Chelate 50mg daily 4. Kelp or seaweed preparations

Footnote: These are suggested schedules only and your doctor may vary them to suit your particular case.
FOR PRODUCT AVAILABILITY CHART SEE PAGES 144-145.

Side effects can usually be avoided if the dosage of Androcur is reduced. Once your skin is looking good, the dose can be reduced way down to say 2.5 to 5mg daily when side effects should disappear. In the long term the lowest possible dose that can keep your skin looking good should be used and your own doctor can guide you on this. (See Table 6). Androcur is available on an authority prescription for women suffering with the effects of excessive male hormones and in such cases, is not expensive.

Aldactone

The chemical name for Aldactone is spironolactone and, like Androcur, this is a drug with a dual action being not only a diuretic but also an effective anti-male hormone. Aldactone is not as powerful in its anti-male hormone effect as Androcur, but may be sufficient for some women with facial hair, acne or balding. It is often preferable to use Aldactone rather than Androcur in women with obesity, high blood pressure, fluid retention, severe depression, or in older women who smoke or who are unable to tolerate the oral contraceptive pill.

The amount needed to control acne and facial hair varies between different women. (See Table 6). If breakthrough bleeding occurs or if contraception is required, Aldactone can be taken with the oral contraceptive pill. You must not become pregnant while taking Aldactone as, like Androcur, it may cause feminisation of the developing male foetus.

Aldactone may cause minor side effects such as breakthrough bleeding, slight breast enlargement, nausea, muscle cramps and an imbalance in potassium levels, but these may be avoided by reducing the dose.

Other Hormonal Treatments

In some women with mild acne and/or facial hair, a very good result can be obtained simply by taking the **female hormone oestrogen**. This will reduce the production of male hormones from the ovary and reduce production of oily secretions from the skin's sebaceous glands. In women with a uterus it is also necessary to give progestogen to regulate menstrual bleeding and only progestogens without male (androgenic) properties should be used. Many of today's oral contraceptive pills contain androgenic progestogens and these should be avoided as they may worsen acne and facial hair. Your doctor can tailor-make an oral contraceptive pill for you containing oestrogen and a non-androgenic progestogen such as Provera, Duphaston, or ideally, Androcur.

In Europe, Australia and New Zealand, women have the benefit of commercially available oral contraceptive pills containing oestrogen and non-androgenic progestogens such as Desogestrel or Androcur. These types of feminine oral contraceptive pills will usually cure acne and improve skin texture.

102

Menopausal and post-menopausal women with facial hair often find that the natural oestrogen in their **hormone replacement therapy** greatly reduces this problem, especially if a small dose of Androcur or Aldactone is added.

Excessive male hormone production from the adrenal glands can be suppressed by taking a very small dose of a **cortisone-type preparation** such as dexamethasone once a night upon retiring. One should use only the smallest possible dose of cortisone-type drugs as an impaired response to stress may occur.

The Story of Julia

Timely hormonal therapy may help to avoid unnecessary surgery as was the case for Julia, a 32-year-old woman who came to see me complaining of symptoms typical of **polycystic ovarian disorder**. Since the birth of her son eight years ago, she had developed PMT, facial hair and acne. Julia had bouts of sharp pelvic pains and an ultrasound scan of her pelvis revealed enlarged ovaries with many small cysts around their periphery. She had consulted a surgeon who told her that the only option was to remove her left ovary and take a wedge of tissue out of her right ovary. Julia was alarmed at this prospect because she did not want to lose an ovary this early in life. She consulted another doctor who prescribed a low-dose oral contraceptive pill, but unfortunately it contained an androgenic progestogen and did not help her facial hair and acne. We discussed the possibility of suppressing her androgen producing ovarian cysts with oestrogen and Androcur and she was delighted to learn that Androcur would cure her acne and facial hair. I prescribed Estigyn .05mg daily and Androcur 50mg for two weeks every month and advised her to avoid surgery as her ovarian cysts were typical of polycystic ovaries and not a tumour or cancer. After six months of Estigyn and Androcur, Julia's ovaries had returned to their normal size, their cysts had become much smaller and her skin was clear and much more feminine in appearance. Julia also found the treatment very convenient as it provided her with reliable contraception.

The Story of Barbara

Excessive secretion of male hormones associated with **polycystic ovaries** is quite common and can be responsible for much suffering and confusion which was exactly the case for 34-year-old Barbara who had been trying to become pregnant for more than two years. Barbara's menstrual cycle had always been infrequent and irregular and every three to four months she would have a menstrual flow that was heralded by PMT, large blind pimples and depression. Since the age of 18, she had developed facial hair and gradually gained excessive weight. Her mother said it was all the fault of her diet and that if she gave up fats and sugars her pimples would clear. Barbara's mother's surprise was only surpassed by Barbara's relief when I explained that her problems were due to excessive levels of male hormones.

I referred Barbara to an infertility specialist so that she could receive fertility drugs to stimulate regular ovulation in her polycystic ovaries. Barbara became pregnant with the fertility drugs and nine months after the birth of her daughter, came to see me as her polycystic ovaries were once again over-producing male hormones. Subsequently, Barbara's facial hair and acne were very well controlled with Estigyn and Androcur and a weight-loss programme.

The Story of Susan

Susan, an actress, comedienne and singer was understandably very concerned with keeping her skin at its best. In her early 30s her hormonal balance changed after having had three children, and she developed "**mature aged acne**".

She became quite obsessed when every month before her period several blind pimples would appear on her chin and forehead and her husband and children complained to me that she sounded like a broken record. In her eyes, the pimples were like volcanos and she resorted to wearing bandaids on her face to conceal them. Her family and friends could hardly see these few pimples and told her that she was being overly anxious.

I referred Susan to a hormone specialist (endocrinologist) who began her on Aldactone tablets. These helped her acne but caused annoying breakthrough bleeding. Her specialist then tried Androcur and oestrogen tablets, but Susan was not able to tolerate oestrogen in oral (tablet) form as it caused nausea.

Her endocrinologist was by this time understanding that actresses are highly strung and sensitive creatures and racked his brains for an alternative to facial bandaids.

He suggested to Susan that she try oestrogen in injection form and so she began a course of monthly Primogyn Depot injections, each one being given at the end of her menstrual bleeding. Much to the relief of the doctor and Susan's family, this stopped the mild acne and she stopped wearing bandaids on her beautiful face.

It may seem minor to you but it is another example of how only a minor imbalance in the ratio of female to male hormones can cause small or large physical changes that in an individual can have ruinous effects.

For women who over-produce male hormones, therapy with oestrogen and anti-male hormones can be dramatically effective. These treatments are slow acting with nine to twelve months of therapy being needed for a total relief of symptoms. However, it is not a cure and symptoms such as acne, hirsutism or balding usually return if hormonal therapy is stopped. For permanent control, it is usually necessary to continue treatment on a long-term basis with interruption if pregnancy is desired.

These hormonal treatments should not be started before the sexual development and longitudinal growth spurt of adolescence is completed, otherwise a reduction in the attainment of height may occur. Furthermore, therapy needs to be guided under strict medical supervision and regular blood tests.

THE THYROID GLAND

The thyroid gland is the soft fleshy mound in front of the Adam's apple. Underactivity of this gland is not an uncommon cause of unpleasant changes in appearance and demeanour in middle-aged to elderly women. An underactive thyroid gland produces insufficient amounts of thyroid hormones and this imbalance may occur slowly and insidiously over a period of years. **Thyroid hormone controls the metabolic rate of the cells,** meaning the rate at which the cells burn up nutrients to produce energy for vital body processes. Thus insufficient thyroid hormone may cause you to gain weight without overeating, and your level of activity may diminish with a slowness in your speech, reflexes and mental activity. Your body temperature and pulse rate may decrease, your voice may deepen and constipation may set in. Without thyroid hormone, your face becomes puffy, your skin thickened and dry and your scalp hair and eyebrows become sparser.

Because these changes usually occur very gradually, they may not be recognised as a medical problem and simply seen as a sign of getting older or the menopause. If you notice any such changes, ask your doctor for a blood test to measure your blood levels of thyroid hormone and the function of your thyroid gland. Thankfully, all the unpleasant and unsightly changes of an underactive thyroid gland can be reversed by taking a daily replacement tablet of thyroid hormone.

Some doctors believe in the concept of resistance to thyroid hormone which means that your body cells become unresponsive to normal amounts of thyroid hormone. Women with thyroid resistance complain of tiredness and excessive weight and yet their blood tests for levels of thyroid hormone are normal and in rare cases may be even greater than normal. In such cases supplemental doses of thyroid hormone have been tried, but this is not without danger as too much thyroid hormone can strain the heart and increase the risk of osteoporosis. Women receiving thyroid hormone tablets need to be carefully monitored by their doctor to keep their blood levels within the normal range.

In women who are obese because of thyroid resistance, special tests to measure the metabolic rate can be done by a hormone specialist (endocrinologist). If the metabolic rate is low, extra thyroid hormone tablets are given to increase the metabolic rate back into the normal range, when weight loss should occur.

There are two types of thyroid hormone — Thyroxine or T4 and Tertroxin or T3. In the body T4 is converted to T3 which is the more active and potent form of thyroid hormone.

If you have an underactive thyroid gland and do not feel well or are unable to lose weight by taking Thyroxine (T4) tablets, you could ask your doctor about the possibility of changing to, or supplementing with Tertroxin (T3) tablets. Logically, T3 tablets are likely to be more effective in women with a poor response to T4 tablets, because T3 has a more rapid and powerful effect on your metabolism. Tertroxin (T3) tablets are not more expensive than Thyroxine (T4) tablets, but they must be given two or three times daily. The starting dose of Tertroxin is around 5 micrograms (mcg), three times daily with a gradual increase to around 20 to 60mcg daily. Your doctor can tailor-make the dosage for you to keep you feeling and looking good and to maintain your blood tests within the normal range.

THE ADRENAL GLAND

We have seen that overactive adrenal glands could make us hairy and masculine in appearance. These same adrenals could have even more devastating effects upon the appearance if they over-produce the hormone cortisone. **Excessive adrenal gland production of cortisone results in "Cushings Syndrome" causing a rare but horrible collection of physical changes.** As with most hormonal disorders, the physical changes appear gradually and may be mistakenly attributed to diet, lifestyle or age.

In Cushings Syndrome, changes to the physique can make it resemble an "orange on toothpicks" with a fat trunk, a "buffalo hump" at the back of the neck, a round moon-shaped face and skinny muscle-wasted limbs! The skin may also be affected and becomes thin with purple stretch marks and increased bruising and facial hair.

The most common cause of Cushings Syndrome is the long-term administration of cortisone tablets to treat conditions such as severe arthritis or asthma and so doctors always try to give their patients the smallest possible dose of these life-saving drugs. Cushings Syndrome may also occur because of a tumour of the pituitary or adrenal gland.

The amount of cortisone produced by your adrenal glands is easily checked with blood and urine tests. If a tumour of the pituitary or adrenal gland is discovered, surgical treatment is required.

THE PITUITARY GLAND

The pituitary gland may cause major changes in the appearance if it over-produces **growth hormone** in adult life after normal growth has ceased. This is not a common occurrence which is fortunate as the effects of excessive growth hormone on the skull, feet and hands may enlarge them considerably requiring a change in the size of hats, gloves and shoes. The length of the bones will not increase, but the soft tissues of the body and cartilage of the joints will enlarge causing an increase in the size of the jaw and nose so that the face will eventually assume a coarse, heavy-featured look with a protruding jaw line.

The physical condition caused by excessive growth hormone is called Acromegaly. Because these changes occur slowly, once again they may be mistakenly put down to overeating or getting older, especially as Acromegaly is uncommon.

The cause of this condition is usually a tumour of the pituitary gland which could be cured by surgery.

Cushings Syndrome and Acromegaly are awful diseases but, luckily, they are the rare and extreme cases — the most terrible results of how hormones can affect your appearance.

CHAPTER 9

HOW YOUR HORMONES AFFECT YOUR WEIGHT

Many overweight women choose to believe that their excessive weight may be due to glandular disorders such as imbalances in the thyroid or adrenal glands, but in reality less than one in a hundred overweight persons should be blaming their glands. Some of these women go to a hormone specialist (endocrinologist) in search of such a glandular cause and this is often a frustrating experience because if you are obese and otherwise well, it is unlikely that your glands are at fault.

Most women who are obese, become that way simply because they take in more energy in the form of calories or kilojoules (4.2 kilojoules = 1 calorie) than the amount of energy they spend in maintaining and exercising the body. You require about 1,000 to 1,500 calories every 24 hours just to maintain internal bodily functions, with the exact number of needed calories determined by your metabolic rate. Those with a slow metabolic rate have a higher chance of obesity and often complain that the mere sight or smell of food adds a few extra fat cells. Conversely, those with a high metabolic rate can often eat high calorie foods with impunity and remain alluringly svelte.

THE METABOLIC RATE

The metabolic rate of an individual appears to be the most important determinant of body type and weight. Conventional medical texts tell us that metabolic rate is determined by several factors, namely:

1. The function of your thyroid gland;

2. Your genetic inheritance;

3. The amount of exercise you do as exercise increases the metabolic rate;

4. Your personality type or how you respond to stress. In hyperactive people, stress increases the activity of the sympathetic nervous system which releases adrenalin and increases body heat production. This causes more calories to be burnt and switches off the appetite. In easy-going or more phlegmatic types, stress seems to act on the hypothalamus in the opposite way, stimulating the appetite control centre and increasing the intake of calories which causes weight gain. Many obese women will relate to this and find themselves always snacking as a means of coping with stress;

5. The number of calories you consume daily. A low calorie diet lowers the metabolic rate.

YOUR BODY TYPE

The distribution of your fat and your body shape is not determined by your metabolic rate alone. Several experts have determined that **weight and body shape depends on a complex interaction between the major glands of the body**.

Endocrinologist, Dr. Ian Caterson, says that there are basically two body types, namely "android" and "gynaeoid". Caterson says that the "android woman" is obese in the upper part of the body with fat accumulating on the abdomen, chest, neck and arms. The android woman tends to produce excessive amounts of male hormones and is often more masculine in appearance. Android or upper body obesity is not desirable as it is associated with a higher incidence of the medical complications of obesity such as cardiovascular disease, high blood pressure, high cholesterol and diabetes and is the more dangerous type of obesity.

The second body type or "gynaeoid-woman" has an accumulation of fat in the lower half of the body on the buttocks, pelvis, hips and thighs and, according to Caterson, this type of obesity is determined by female hormones. She becomes the epitome of feminism with voluptuous and cuddly curves. Lower body obesity is safer than upper body obesity as it is associated with a lower incidence of high cholesterol, high blood pressure and diabetes.

An American weight expert Dr. Elliot Abravanel adds to Caterson's "Android" and "Gynaeoid" types two other body types — the "thyroid" and "pituitary" types. (Reference 1.) Dr. Abravanel's theories are not widely accepted by the orthodox medical fraternity, but I believe that the four body types he describes have much practical value. In my day-to-day practise of medicine, I can relate to his theory as, generally speaking, my patients fall into one of the four body types he describes.

THE FOUR BODY TYPES

As an exercise, envision yourself as one of the following four types of physique. You can practise fitting your friends and family members into one of these categories.

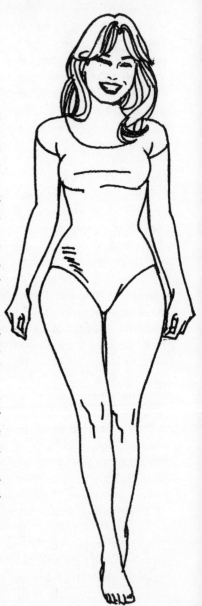

The Gynaeoid Type

In the gynaeoid type of woman, the sex glands (ovaries) and their secreted female hormones have the most influence on body shape and fat distribution. Excessive weight is distributed in feminine areas such as buttocks, pelvis, hips, thighs and breasts. It is unfortunate that this type of fatty tissue may become uneven and lumpy resulting in cellulite.

The typical gynaeoid woman craves fatty foods and spices which stimulate her ovaries to produce even more oestrogen to exaggerate her body shape.

To correct the metabolic imbalance in the gynaeoid woman, it is necessary to establish a diet that does not stimulate the ovaries, but instead stimulates the thyroid and adrenal glands. (See Table 7 on Page 114).

The gynaeoid type of woman may be worried that if she loses her excessive pounds, her sexuality may diminish, but this is not true; the increased energy and wellbeing of a normal body weight can only enhance sexuality.

Gynaeoid women need to stay with their ideal diet for life as of all types of fat, lower body fat is hardest to lose.

The Android Type

The classical android woman is square-shaped with a solid, thick big-boned frame and she is athletic and powerful in appearance. Obesity tends to give her a more masculine appearance. Excessive fat accumulates on the trunk, neck and abdomen causing the stomach to protrude and the waistline to disappear.

If you are an android woman, you will usually be energetic and strong with good staying power when others about you need a coffee break. You have a tendency to overproduce male hormones and may be told you take after your dad.

Android types are definitely not sugarholics or ''sweet tooths'', but instead crave foods high in cholesterol and salt that stimulate their adrenal glands to pump out more steroid hormones. These steroid hormones increase the appetite and unfortunately promote further accumulation of fat and muscle and more masculine features.

To restore metabolic balance in android types, it is necessary to avoid high cholesterol and salty foods. (See Table 8.)

Dr. Caterson suggests that in android types weight loss can be easier and more effective if the excess of male hormones is corrected first. This can be done with hormone therapy. (See Page 101). As the android type loses weight, her production of male hormones will diminish and she will regain a more feminine physique.

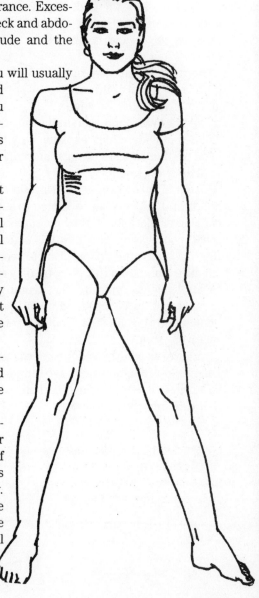

The Thyroid Type

The thyroid type resembles the thoroughbred racehorse with long, fine-boned limbs and a slender neck and can be described as lean and rangy. They lack the enduring stamina of the android types and crave stimulants such as caffeine, sugar and cigarettes for a burst of energy.

Because their thyroid gland is the dominant gland, they have a high metabolic rate and generally burn up calories quickly which explains why they need frequent snacks of sugar and caffeine to keep them going.

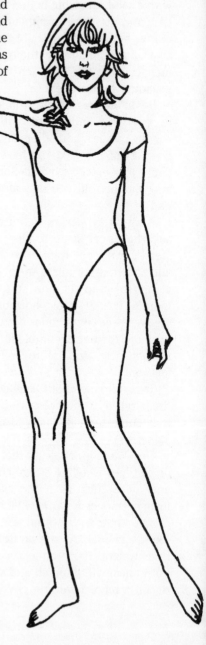

Thyroid types can be excessive in their habits and may become addicted to sugar, caffeine or diet pills. If they continue with these poor eating and lifestyle patterns, they may cause the thyroid gland to become exhausted and from this point on they start to gain weight. Typically, the weight gain is rapid and fat is deposited upon the abdomen and thighs while the limbs remain relatively slim.

An overweight thyroid type needs to rebalance her metabolism by avoiding sugar, soft drinks, sweets, refined carbohydrates and caffeine. (See Table 9.)

The Pituitary Type

The pituitary type is the epitome of the cuddly baby doll type who has never lost her baby fat. She is round all over with a round shaped face and may have a relatively large head. Her limbs, hands and feet are chubby and she has a layer of fat over her chest, although the breasts may not be unduly large.

The typical pituitary type of woman craves dairy products such as cheeses, yoghurt, cream, ice cream, butter and milk. Dr. Abravanel's theory, although unproven, is that dairy products are stimulants to the pituitary gland because they contain the hormone prolactin. To find the ideal diet to restore metabolic balance and promote weight loss in the pituitary type, see Table 10.

The pituitary type is also known as the lymphatic type because she is prone to congestion of her lymphatic system. The lymphatic system is a network of tiny tubes in the subcutaneous layer under the skin that carries fluid and fat away from the limbs. Congestion of the lymphatic system causes fluid retention and puffiness in the limbs.

For further details of the Body Shaping Diet see page 153.

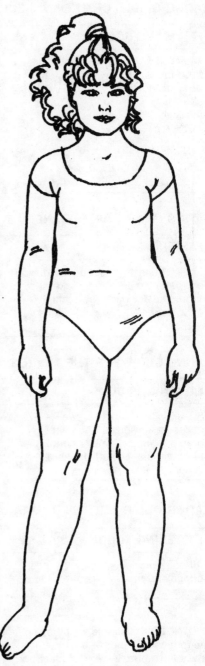

113

EATING GUIDE FOR THE GYNAEOID WOMAN — TABLE 7

FATTENING FOODS	SLIMMING FOODS
Fatty foods, take-away foods, all fried foods, creamy foods, full-fat dairy products, greasy meals, chocolate, spicy foods e.g. Indian, Mexican, Thai foods.	Complex carbohydrates, grains, legumes, seeds, wholemeal cereals, wholemeal bread, low fat dairy products, vegetables, fruits, low fat meat and poultry, all seafoods, eggs, herbs, aromatic salad vegetables and seaweeds can be used to enhance flavours. Some caffeine is allowed — say 2 to 3 cups of coffee daily.

EATING GUIDE FOR THE ANDROID WOMAN — TABLE 8

FATTENING FOODS	SLIMMING FOODS
Eggs, shellfish, coconut, fried foods and fatty greasy foods, take away foods, full-fat dairy products, chocolate, salt and salty foods.	Fish, low fat poultry, vegetables, fruits, grains, nuts, seeds, legumes, wholemeal cereals and bread, low-fat dairy products, low-fat red meat can be eaten 2 to 3 times per week.

EATING GUIDE FOR THE THYROID WOMAN — TABLE 9

FATTENING FOODS	SLIMMING FOODS
Sugar, lollies, candies, sweets, sweet cakes and biscuits, chocolate, honey, jams, caffeine, alcohol, diet pills, stimulants, soft drinks e.g. coke, fanta, pepsi.	Lean meats, all seafoods, poultry, dairy products, eggs, grains, nuts, seeds, wholemeal cereals and bread, vegetables, fruit — only two pieces daily.

EATING GUIDE FOR THE PITUITARY WOMAN — TABLE 10

FATTENING FOODS	SLIMMING FOODS
All dairy products, creamy foods, chocolate, fried foods, fatty foods, take-away foods, greasy foods.	Vegetables, lean meats, organ meats, poultry, seafoods, grains, nuts, seeds, legumes, wholemeal cereals and bread. All fruits.

FOOTNOTE: If you avoid the fattening foods for your own body type you will rebalance the four body glands — the pituitary, thyroid, adrenal and gonads (ovaries) and thus promote the attainment of ideal body weight and body shape.

114

THE SIGNIFICANCE OF BEING OVERWEIGHT

In scientific terms, the body shape or weight alone, cannot be isolated as it is the relationship of body weight to body height that is important. This can be expressed as your "Body Mass Index" (BMI — see glossary), and also in a graph illustrating your weight-for-height. (See Diagram 19). Plot yourself in the weight-for-height graph and you may be surprised.

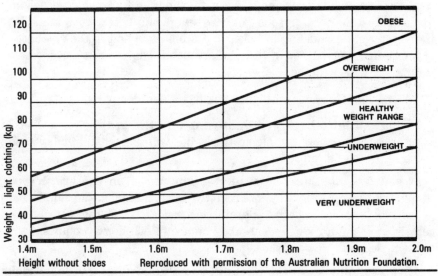

WEIGHT FOR HEIGHT (Use this chart to plot weight and progress)

Weight in light clothing (kg)

Height without shoes   Reproduced with permission of the Australian Nutrition Foundation.

DIAGRAM 19

If you fall in the obese range of the graph you may be subject to the following medical risks:

1. High blood pressure and cardiovascular disease;

2. Diabetes;

3. Respiratory problems;

4. Gall stones;

5. Complicated pregnancies;

6. Arthritis;

7. Cancer of the breast, uterus, gall bladder and bowel. The oestrogen sensitive tumours of the breast and uterus are increased because obese women produce excessive oestrogen;

8. Hormonal and gynaecological disorders such as fibroids and heavy painful periods. Obesity will cause a woman to make more oestrogen in her fatty tissues and this stimulates the growth of fibroids, and may worsen endometriosis and increase menstrual blood flow and pain. As women get fatter their level of the male hormone testosterone increases which increases the tendency to facial hair, greasy skin and acne. Weight loss will improve these gynaecological and skin problems.

9. Sleep apnoea which is the medical term for failure to breathe during sleep. This affects the hypothalamus and reduces oxygen supply to the cells which reduces the metabolic rate and makes it much harder for you to lose weight. Sleep apnoea in obese persons can have severe effects causing a reduction in testosterone production in males and a big reduction in the amount of growth hormone produced by the pituitary gland. These effects may increase the rate at which the body ages;

10. A shorter life span and higher risk of sudden death.

If you fall into the overweight range on the graph, you will also be subject to the above ten medical risks but with less susceptibility than those in the obese range.

If you fall into the very underweight range on the graph, you should try to gain weight by increasing your consumption of calories and protein foods to increase fat and muscle tissues. Try to eat more bread, cereals, grains, nuts, wholemeal cakes, honey, full fat dairy products, eggs, chicken, seafoods and lean meats.

If you remain very underweight, you will be at an increased risk of the following disorders:

1. Low levels of oestrogen with an associated higher risk of osteoporosis and cardiovascular disease;

2. Reduced fertility;

3. Complicated pregnancies.

By understanding your weight-for-height ratio, your body type and the factors that determine your metabolic rate, you are now in a powerful position to change the things that prevent you from achieving the healthy weight range depicted on our graph.

Reference
1. Dr. E. Abravanel *Body Type Diet Book,* Bantam Books

CHAPTER 10

THE MALE MENOPAUSE – FACT OR FICTION?

This chapter is designed for you and your partner if he has a midlife crisis.

The word "menopause" literally means the cessation of menstrual bleeding. In females it signifies that the biological clock has stopped and infertility sets in accompanied by dramatic hormonal changes. So, the word "menopause" cannot apply to men. Yet, even though they seem to be on easy street compared to women, it is indeed a fact that men also are vulnerable to fundamental emotional, mental and physical changes at about 50 years of age and beyond and when Hormone Replacement Therapy (HRT) may be of help to men as well as women.

The first semblance of Hormone Replacement Therapy (HRT) was used on a man in 1889, when a famous neurophysiologist Charles-Edouard Brown-Sequard, gave himself an extract of animal testicles. In his own words this produced "a return of vigour, youthful appetites and desires" due to the male hormone testosterone contained in the animal testicles.

Hormonal Changes In Men

Testosterone production from the testicles is at its peak during the 20s and 30s, and thereafter a slow decline occurs which becomes more pertinent after the age of 50. Despite this, there is a large variation between individual males so that some men at 50 may produce such low levels of testosterone that they no longer feel any inclination to have a sex life, whereas others at 80, have high testosterone levels and are still sexually vigorous. As you are reading this you are probably wondering how you (if you are male) or your partner can be one of the lucky ones and nurture those testicles all the way along throughout life. The ability to produce testosterone is partly genetic so that in many cases it's "like father, like son". We also know that lifestyle plays a role and men who smoke and/or drink alcohol excessively will have lower levels of testosterone in their blood.

As a man ages, not only does the production of testosterone diminish, but so does the ability of his tissues and cells to respond to testosterone. It is a simple matter for a man to see if his testosterone production is down by asking for a blood test.

117

A deficiency of testosterone would be obvious if the blood level was below 8nmol/L, the normal range of testosterone in the blood being 11 to 37 nmol/L. This would be further corroborated by high blood levels of the pituitary hormone called Luteinising Hormone (LH) which is indicative that the pituitary gland is trying to stimulate the sluggish testicles. This blood test could be repeated on three separate occasions, at eight-weekly intervals to demonstrate any trends before deciding if male HRT is needed.

The Symptoms of Testosterone Deficiency
Testosterone deficiency shows up in:
1. Reduced libido, fatigue and behaviourial changes;
2. Shrinkage (atrophy) of the muscles, testicles and penis and softening of the testicles;
3. Reduced rate of growth of facial and body hair;
4. Reduction in virility and ability to achieve orgasm. In severe cases, impotence.

A male who has previously had high levels of testosterone may find that the decreasing testosterone levels that can begin to occur after the age of 50 produce subtle mental and physical changes even though his blood test reveals that his testosterone levels are still within the normal physiological range of 11 to 37 nmol/L. This is because his testosterone levels are much lower than they used to be and he is sensitive to the decreasing levels.

Subtle changes of decreasing testosterone production may range from depression, loss of confidence, loss of drive and aggression and loss of competitiveness in all spheres. The warrior man finds himself becoming a bit of a mouse. If such a male takes himself along to the doctor he may be told that all this is symptomatic of the psychological male midlife crisis, especially after a full physical checkup fails to reveal any medical problems. He may be told that this crisis is due to a plateau in his career, looming retirement, unrealised ambitions, getting older, overdoing it, or stress.

He may be offered a course of anti-depressants, sedatives or tranquillisers and referred for counselling to assuage his growing self-doubts. Men are more reluctant than women to accept a course of such therapy preferring to numb their anxieties at the bar with their mates. Unfortunately, alcohol ingestion, if it becomes regular or excessive, often further reduces the production of testosterone leading to an aggravation of the mental and physical imbalance.

It is vital to check the possibility of a hormonal contribution and, if this is suspected, a short trial of hormone replacement therapy with testosterone can be tried.

HORMONE REPLACEMENT THERAPY (HRT) FOR MEN

Oral Androgens

The word "androgen" is the medical term for "male hormone".

Androgens may be given on a regular basis in tablet (oral) form. Some common brands are Testomet (methyltestosterone) or the relatively new Andriol (testosterone undecanoate). There is a possible link between Testomet and liver cancer and Andriol can produce nausea if taken in large doses.

Proviron (mesterolone) is another brand of oral androgen but many men find it as ineffective, as a placebo.

All in all, oral androgens often prove to be unsatisfactory in their effect and a significant proportion of men with severe testosterone deficiency complain that oral testosterone is not effective. It may not be wise to use oral androgens as an introductory trial in a middle-aged man who has a subtle androgen deficiency, and who is wondering whether male hormone replacement therapy holds the key to wellbeing. If oral androgens are ineffectual, a negative value judgement against all other forms of male HRT may be made, with further attempts being rejected.

Androgen Injections

If a man is considering a short-term trial of male HRT there is probably no more definitive way of proving or disproving its benefit than with a three to four month course of monthly injections of androgen. If a deficiency of testosterone is responsible for the mental, physical and sexual fatigue of middle-age, then the androgen injection should greatly reduce, if not abolish these symptoms within one to two weeks. This brings a great sense of relief and apart from the alleviation of symptoms, the androgen injections can produce a feeling of great energy, vitality and can be a superb anti-depressant.

Suitable androgen injections are Primoteston Depot (testosterone oenanthate) or Sustanon (testosterone propionate), which can be given as a deep oily intramuscular injection into the buttocks each month for three to four months. A follow-up appointment with the doctor should be made two months after the final injection, by which time their effect would no longer be apparent. During this consultation, a decision to abandon or continue with testosterone replacement therapy in the long term can be made. **If a patient decides to continue with testosterone replacement for several years or decades, the most effective way in which to deliver the testosterone to the tissues would be through a hormone implant.**

Androgen Implants

Each implant contains 200mg of testosterone and if three of these are inserted at once, they will provide good blood levels of testosterone for six months. The implants are buried into the fat of the abdominal wall or buttocks. (See Page 90). Most men find these implants very effective and free of side effects. This is understandable as the testosterone is absorbed from the implant directly into the blood, bypassing the liver and carried to the receptive tissues and organs.

Side-Effects Of Androgen Replacement Therapy

If testosterone is given in any form, be it tablets, injections or implants on a long-term basis, it needs to be carefully supervised by a doctor. Testosterone replacement therapy given over several to many years may cause problems and the tablet forms are probably more likely to do this than are the other forms. **Ideally, the lowest dose of testosterone should be used to maintain a good quality of mental, physical and sexual wellbeing.**

Your partner should be made aware that testosterone replacement therapy can increase the size of the prostate gland. The prostate gland is situated at the neck of the bladder and secretes fluid to add to the sperm during ejaculation. If it becomes enlarged, difficulties may be experienced during the passage of urine with such symptoms as difficulty in beginning urination, dribbling after passing urine, slowness and delay in completing urination and urinary frequency occurring. If these problems persist, surgical removal of the prostate gland may be required. Long-term testosterone replacement therapy may also increase the risk of cancer of the prostate gland. If testosterone doses are excessive, they may produce an unfavourable influence on blood cholesterol patterns thus increasing the risk of cardiovascular disease. Excessive doses may also produce an abnormally high level of red blood cells (poly-cythaemia).

Overall, **testosterone replacement therapy is safe and can be of tremendous value provided it is given by an expert in the field and followed up by annual checkups from a urologist.**

Can The Male Menopause Cause Impotence?

Minor degrees of testosterone deficiency do not cause impotence and the level of testosterone deficiency would need to be marked before inability to achieve erection and orgasm occurred. Most men presenting to the doctor with impotence at the time of midlife do not have a significant testosterone deficiency.

Other factors such as general fitness, cardiovascular status, long-term abuse of cigarettes and alcohol, various medications, stress and loss of confidence are more likely to cause impotence especially if these factors occur in combination. Most impotent men have a functional disorder of the "spongy" or erectile tissue in the penis. This erectile tissue is called the corpus cavernosum and during a normal erection it becomes congested with blood. In impotent men this congestion does not occur and so the penis remains small and soft. New treatments available for this problem are vasoactive drugs (Prostin, Prostaglandin E, Alprostadil) that can be self-injected into the erectile tissue of the penis when required. These injections enable the male to regain control of his erections even though he is using artificial means and most users of this method are very satisfied. If this fails, penile implants can be successful. The reader who wishes to know more about male impotence is referred to an excellent and comprehensive book entitled *It's Up To You* written by Warwick Williams, published by Williams & Wilkins, Adis Pty Ltd.

Female Hormones For Men

It used to be thought that the prime female hormone oestrogen exerted its effects only upon female sexual organs such as the vagina, uterus and breasts. We now know that oestrogen exerts profound and widespread effects upon many other tissues, such as the brain, liver, bones, joints, skin, heart and arteries. In particular, oestrogen has a very favourable effect on blood cholesterol as it helps the enzymes that break down cholesterol and thus reduces the chances of our blood vessels becoming blocked with fatty hard plaques of cholesterol. In the long term, oestrogen helps to reduce diseases of the heart and blood vessels.

This observation has led some of our modern-day scientists to come up with the hypothesis that if we give natural oestrogen to males we can reduce their current high rate of cardiovascular disease. Indeed, there are now clinical trials under way to see if giving natural oestrogen to males between the ages of 30 and 60 will reduce their cholesterol levels and rate of heart attacks. Oestrogen may also reduce the rate of cancer of the prostate gland so there could be several ways whereby oestrogen could give men an extra ten years or so of life.

All is not roses, however, as oestrogen being a potent female hormone is likely to exert some possibly undesirable side-effects in our virile male species. These could include breast tenderness, loss of sex drive, impotence and reduced sperm production.

NUTRITIONAL STRATEGIES FOR THE MALE MENOPAUSE

Diet and lifestyle are supremely important for the male finding himself with reduced mental and sexual performance during midlife.

Exercise is vitally important, but I believe, given our current high rate of male cardiovascular disease, that all men should undergo a cardiac stress test (exercise ECG) before initiating an increase in their exercise programme. A good age to have a cardiac stress test is 50 years, or even at 40 years if there is a poor family history.

Some specific nutritional supplements can be tried and these offer a useful alternative to those men who do not feel comfortable about Hormone Replacement Therapy.

NATURAL MALE MENOPAUSE KIT

SUPPLEMENT	DOSE	ROLE
Vitamin E	500 iu daily	Anti-oxidant action, protects cell structures and reduces oxidative damage to lining of blood vessels. Increases efficiency of oxygen utilisation by cardiac muscle.
Minerals Zinc Selenium Manganese	100 mg daily 50 mcg daily 5 mg daily	Catalysts for enzyme systems thereby increasing metabolic efficiency. Anti-oxidant action.
Ginseng	500mg, 3 times daily	Ancient "glandular tonic" used by Chinese and Russian civilisations. Acts as a general tonic.
Hi B Complex Tablet	1 daily	Necessary for efficient function of central and peripheral nervous system. Excellent if under stress/alcohol excess.

MALE MIDLIFE CRISIS

Technically, we know that men cannot go through a literal menopause. However, for many men the phase of midlife brings significant hormonal changes and important physical and psychological changes. Put these all together in a melting pot and you may very well have the ingredients for a male midlife crisis. This is undoubtedly one of the reasons why divorce rates soar at this time and many women get the shock of their lives. These women are left in the well known "empty nest syndrome" with hubby fleeing the familiar domestic scene. Conversely, the male not infrequently gets the "nesting syndrome" and spreads his wings with a younger woman finding that her youthfulness rekindles his feelings of manliness and passion and he feels that life is beginning all over again.

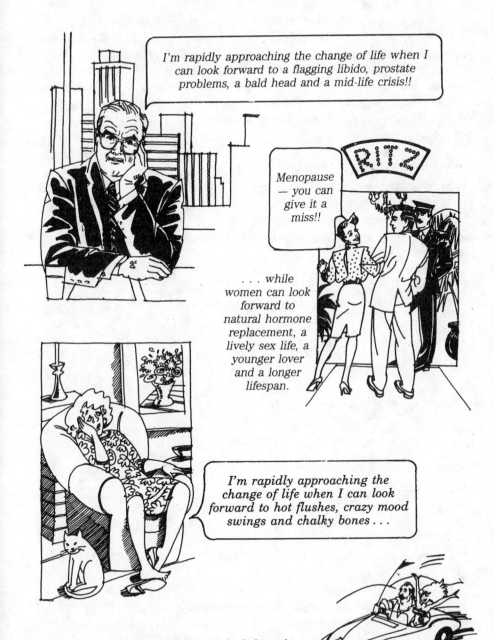

This situation is very emotive and can be extremely traumatic in the short and long term. It could probably be averted in many cases if males received more information and supportive counselling especially with their wives at this time in their lives. In some cases, the timely use of testosterone replacement therapy, even if only on a temporary basis, can bring back the sparkle into a long-term sexual relationship.

If older men keep running off with younger women, what will the women they leave behind do? Well, one obvious strategy is that these women can also get the "nesting syndrome" and run off with younger men! I see quite a few older women doing this and find it an interesting sociological phenomenon. Anyway, there are statistics to support such behaviour, as menopausal women who take natural oestrogen have been found, on average, to live nine to ten years longer than their male counterparts. To avoid loneliness in old age a man ten years younger could probably fit the bill very nicely!

CHAPTER 11

HOW TO MAINTAIN YOUR SEXUALITY AND IMPROVE A FLAGGING LIBIDO

Thousands of women have written to me over the years revealing their sexual frustrations and problems and it has been a shock to see how little help women receive with these problems.

Ideally, as a woman ages she becomes more relaxed as a sexual being, realising that the most important thing about sex is that it is fun and stress-relieving. She is also more knowledgeable about her own individual needs and what it takes to give her sexual satisfaction. Maturity enables her to be more easily assertive and effective in asking to have her needs fulfilled. Many women have told me that their sexual desire increases as they age and for most of them there is more sexual interest, pleasure and capacity for orgasm. These women confirm that enjoyment of sex appears to rise continuously into the middle years and remains stable from that time on.

That would be great — but it could be wishful thinking. **As a doctor I have found that many women have huge fluctuations in libido (sex drive) and enjoyment of sex especially as they are approaching the menopause.**

When the level of the sex hormones of both male and female variety are low, the sex drive will suffer. This may occur for six to twelve months after childbirth and also gradually after the age of 45 to 50 years as the menopause approaches. If the levels of the sex hormones are low, there may also be a change in the personality and a woman may become disinterested and unresponsive, and shun the advances of the man she has previously loved and desired.

It is sad when these problems in older women disrupt an otherwise good relationship or marriage. This is unnecessary because early help could salvage both the woman's sexuality and the man's ego. Then, divorce rates and the number of lonely middle-aged people would definitely decrease.

It is interesting for me as a doctor to find that poor libido or sex drive is a common problem in women. No one ever complains about having too much libido and indeed it seems for some the more the better!

The greatest destroyers of the libido include:

1. Insufficient production of the male and female sex hormones. This can be aggravated by an unhealthy lifestyle and diet, and laboratory testing shows that men and women who drink and/or smoke excessively have lower levels of sex hormones in their blood. Women who smoke heavily are more prone to an early menopause which will further reduce their libido.

2. In men the fear of poor performance or premature ejaculation causes stress and reduces libido. Thankfully, women are far less prone to this type of stress.

3. Menopausal women are susceptible to vaginal shrinkage and dryness and so may experience pain during sexual intercourse. Furthermore, if shrinkage of the vulva and clitoris occurs, normal lubrication and orgasmic capacity become very difficult. Understandably, many menopausal and post-menopausal women in this situation avoid sexual contact.

4. Various prescription medications may reduce libido. Take the example of Peter, a 44-year-old, aggressive business executive. Despite normal ups and downs in their sixteen years of marriage, he and his wife had never had sexual problems until Peter accepted drug treatment for ulcer pains. Despite his strong desires, he is discouraged to find that his erections no longer last. Or take the case of Christine who has started anti-depressant medication for her chronic depression. Although her moods and libido have returned to normal, she is frustrated by her inability to achieve orgasm. It is now increasingly recognised that situations such as those of Peter and Christine are common. **A wide range of drugs may affect sexual function causing loss of libido, arousal difficulty, orgasmic dysfunction or reproductive impairment.** The most common drugs to cause these problems are appetite suppressants, some muscle relaxants, some drugs for epilepsy, some drugs to prevent headaches, some drugs to treat high blood pressure, some sedatives and anti-depressants, some anti-ulcer drugs and some hormones, particularly anti-male hormones. Make sure you check with your doctor before you're given a new medication as you may be in for a surprise when your sexual ability and desire become reduced through the medication. There is often a suitable alternative drug which will not do this as new derivatives of older drugs which have a lesser incidence of side effects are becoming available every day.

5. Boredom and routine may creep into a long-term relationship, especially if the male partner is unaware of the needs and changes in the sexuality of a woman as she ages. He may not realise that he will need to be gentler and take more time to stimulate his partner before entry.

WHAT TO DO FOR A POOR LIBIDO

If you find yourself in the quandary of poor libido and loss of sexual enjoyment and performance which is disrupting a valuable relationship, see your doctor for a thorough medical checkup to see if there is a physical disorder or disease that could be causing this situation. Such disorders are thyroid imbalance, high blood pressure, diabetes, hardening of the arteries, lower back problems or diseases of the nervous system, such as multiple sclerosis. If, after a thorough physical examination, your doctor cannot find any obvious physical causes to explain your problem, the next step is to have the level of the sex hormones measured in the blood. If these levels are low or borderline (at the lower limit of the normal range), you should benefit greatly from specific Hormone Replacement Therapy.

It may require a little time, patience and experimentation with different types of hormones to find the right combination to turn you on. Some combinations and types of synthetic hormones will frankly turn you off and for this reason women who have been taking the synthetic hormones found in the oral contraceptive pill for some time often experience a reduction in libido. Similarly, some menopausal and pre-menopausal women find that conventional oral HRT with oestrogen and semi-natural progesterones does not recapture their former enjoyment of sex.

GENERAL MEASURES TO HELP A POOR LIBIDO

You and your doctor have several alternatives to play with to encourage the libido and I will qualify these with my own clinical results. Firstly, the use of conventional tablet forms of HRT containing natural oestrogens and semi-natural progesterones will restore the capacity for a normal sex life in the majority of women suffering with a sex hormone deficiency during pre-menopausal, menopausal or post-menopausal years. In addition, for those women with a dry over-sensitive or fragile vagina that fails to lubricate adequately, the use of vaginal oestrogen creams or pessaries applied to the vagina and vaginal lips or vulva can be extremely beneficial. Many women with these problems turn to bland creams or jellies such as 'K-Y jelly', but these have only a temporary lubricating action.

Conversely, hormonal creams and pessaries restore and rejuvenate the mucosal lining of the vagina and vaginal lips and improve the circulation of blood to the clitoral area, thus restoring the capacity for natural lubrication and orgasm (See Diagram 20). Some of my patients have told me that vaginal oestrogen creams or pessaries act like an aphrodisiac and make them feel very sexy.

Some menopausal women have shrinkage of the vagina, vulva and clitoris and painful scar tissue forming in the roof of the vagina which can make

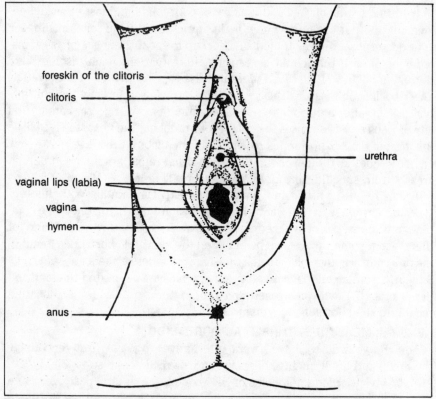

foreskin of the clitoris

clitoris

urethra

vaginal lips (labia)

vagina

hymen

anus

DIAGRAM 20: EXTERNAL GENITALIA OF THE FEMALE (VULVA)

it impossible for the penis to penetrate without pain. These problems can be overcome by regularly massaging the inside of the vaginal walls with **oestrogen cream** and gently stretching apart the vaginal walls with your fingers. This can be done gradually more and more each day and there is no need to stretch excessively and cause pain. In some women, particularly those who have undergone a premature menopause, shrinkage of the vulva and clitoris can be extreme and in these cases, both an oestrogen cream and a **male hormone cream** can be massaged gently into the vulva and clitoris two or three times daily. The chemist can make up the male hormone cream specially from ampoules of pure testosterone which are mixed in a 2 to 5% concentration in oily base. These ampoules are called Primoteston.

In some women the vulva becomes dry and extremely itchy and the lips of the vagina become pale, shrunken and chronically inflamed. In women suffering with such a dry, itchy and inflamed vulva, **naturopathic supple-**

ments can reduce the discomfort and inflammation. The appropriate supplements to take are evening primrose oil capsules, 3000mg daily and the Naudicelle brand of evening primrose oil is particularly beneficial because of its high concentration of gamma linoleic acid (GLA). Natural Vitamin E 500 international units daily should also be taken along with a high quality antioxidant tablet in a dose of one tablet two times daily. Added benefit will be obtained by taking Vitamin C 6000 mg daily either in a powdered or tablet form.

If recurrent infections of the vagina or vulva complicate the problem, bathing the area in tea tree oil shampoo instead of soap is useful. If infection with candida is present, the tea tree oil shampoo will act as a deterrent to the growth of the candida fungus and added effect may be obtained by the application of nystatin cream to the vagina on retiring at night.

HORMONE THERAPY

Some menopausal women experience a total loss of libido, even to the point where they become frigid or cannot tolerate the sexual advances of their partner. In such cases, conventional hormone replacement therapy using oestrogen and progesterone tablets may not be able to overcome the problem satisfactorily. These women may find that **injections of natural female and male sex hormones** produce a return of a healthy libido and increased mental and physical wellbeing. These injections can be very helpful for menopausal women experiencing total loss of libido associated with severe anxiety and depression and are also effective in overcoming loss of libido and depression after a hysterectomy. Injections of natural female and male sex hormones can often overcome fatigue associated with the menopause and post-hysterectomy stage. These injections are oily and need to be given deeply into the muscles of the buttock where they provide a storage or depot of hormones that will be slowly released into the blood for a four to five week period. Thus, the injections will need to be repeated approximately every 5 to 6 weeks.

The natural oestrogen injection is available under the brand name of Primogyn Depot. Natural progesterone injection is available under the name of Proluton Depot and natural male hormone is combined with natural oestrogen in the injection known as Primodian Depot. Your own doctor can try various combinations of these injections until the right dosage and balance is discovered to bring back a healthy libido and sense of mental and physical wellbeing for each individual. **Make sure to check with your doctor that you are receiving injections of the natural types of hormones as the synthetic hormones will not have the desired result.** Another suitable way to administer natural oestrogen and male hormone is in the form of **implants**

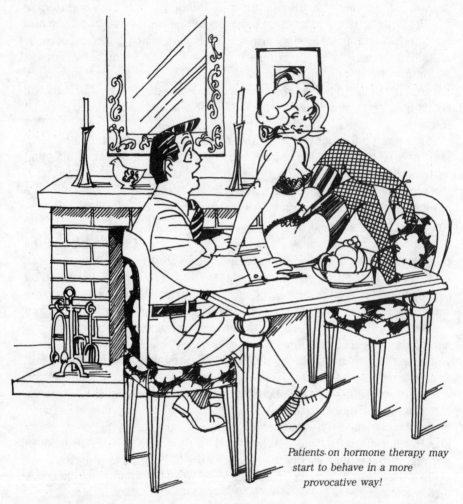

Patients on hormone therapy may start to behave in a more provocative way!

which are small pellets of compressed crystals of hormones. These implants
are about the size of a small pea and are surgically buried into the fat of
the buttocks or abdomen through a very small cut made in the overlying
skin. These implants can be inserted painlessly after anaesthetising the skin
with a local anaesthetic and only one or two stitches will be required to close
the incision after the implant has been inserted. (See Page 90). The hormone pellets will be slowly absorbed from the fat into the blood and will
product a beneficial effect upon libido and sexual wellbeing for a variable
period lasting from three to nine months. After this time another implant
can be inserted if the symptoms of the menopause return. Many women find

that they tolerate injections or implants of natural hormones better than they tolerate hormonal tablets and so they are a valuable alternative to bear in mind.

A healthy sex drive or libido in women is equally dependent upon sufficient amounts of female and male hormones. These days male hormones are being used more and more to complement the replacement of the female hormones, oestrogen and progesterone in menopausal and post-menopausal women. **Natural male hormones may be administered in the form of a testosterone implant or Primodian injection and may be just what's needed to lift a sexual low or crisis.** The physiological effects of male hormones are to increase the size and sensitivity of the clitoris which may have been very tiny, about the size of a match head. There is now increased responsiveness to sexual stimulation, either partner or self-induced. Male hormones may increase the intensity and frequency of orgasms or enable a woman to have an orgasm for the first time in her life. The result can be astonishing and women who have always found sex a bore or a chore may change after two to six weeks and thereafter progression often occurs without further hormone therapy. Sexual pleasure and arousal may set off hormonal changes that are self-perpetuating. Patients on hormone therapy may start to have sexy dreams and dress in a more provocative way.

Many women worry that male hormones will turn them into hairy amazons and are too frightened to try them. If male hormones are used for long periods of time or in excessive dosage, they can cause facial hair, slight weight gain, greasy, pimply skin and sometimes deepening of the voice. Older women may notice a desirable increase in pubic hair. Thankfully, the desired effects of male hormones usually occur before unwanted side effects appear. If male hormones are taken intermittently for no more than three months at a time, these possible side effects should be minimal or non-existent and will only be temporary. It is important that women experiencing menopause or sexual difficulties are made aware of all their options and the possible side effects of treatment. It is important to avoid pregnancy during hormone treatment for sexual problems and for eight weeks after finishing treatment. Some menopausal women become so distressed and depressed by their loss of sexuality and vitality that they are willing to accept minor side effects such as a few extra facial hairs and pimples for the benefit of a course of natural male hormones.

The first widespread recognition of the use of male hormones in Australia appeared in the *Medical Journal of Australia* in 1973, but their clinical use for sexual difficulties remains controversial.

I personally believe that temporary use of natural male hormones in injectible form is extremely useful in the situation where a woman's libido and sexuality is at such a low ebb that she can no longer cope or her marriage is about to collapse. A three to twelve month course of monthly injections containing a combination of natural oestrogen, progesterone and testosterone can be dramatically effective in increasing sexual, mental and emotional wellbeing and pull a woman out of an otherwise endless pit.

Needless to say, it is essential that women undergo these hormonal treatments only under the careful supervision of a doctor who is interested and experienced in women's health. Before any type of Hormone Replacement Therapy, whether it be in the form of tablets, creams, implants or injections, a thorough general checkup and a screening for breast and gynaecological cancer must be painstakingly performed and repeated every 12 months. This is because an early silent cancer of the breast, liver or uterus could be stimulated in growth by hormone replacement therapy.

NUTRITIONAL HELP FOR POOR LIBIDO

Patients often ask me if there is something natural or nutritional they can take to stimulate their flagging libido. Indeed there is, and a **suitable diet** to provide your sex glands with all the raw materials to manufacture sex hormones is one that contains:

- Seafoods (unless you suffer with high cholesterol when intake of crustaceans should be limited);
- Unprocessed grains, nuts, seeds and legumes;
- Raw salads and raw fruits;
- Free range eggs — three to four per week;
- Raw fruit and vegetable juices.

Specific nutritional supplements may also help your sex glands to manufacture hormones and will aid in balancing the biochemistry of the brain centres that are involved with libido and mood control.

These supplements are:

- Vitamin E in natural form in a dosage of 1,000 international units daily;
- B complex vitamin tablet, one daily;
- A zinc supplement, 100 mg daily;
- Evening Primrose Oil, 3000 mg daily;
- Amino acid complex, two tablets daily.

All supplements should be taken at the beginning of meals.

IF AT FIRST YOU DON'T SUCCEED . . .

What if, after a checkup, hormone replacement therapy and natural supplements, the libido is still flagging? Firstly, don't give up prematurely as it may be necessary to try several different combinations of hormones and when the right combination is found it may take two to three months to produce the desired effect.

Secondly, take a look at your lifestyle: has it been basically healthy or are you drinking and smoking your sex glands into an early death?

Thirdly, take a look at the quality of communication between you and your partner. Is it blocked by fear, guilt, or poor self-image and low self-esteem, embarrassment, anger, frustration or other negative emotions? If so, you need to go back to basics and receive some counselling from a professional psychologist or doctor who has a special interest in sexual disorders. Such professionals are called sex therapists and this type of counselling can be combined with counselling from a marriage guidance counsellor, if necessary. Your local doctor should be able to refer you to these professionals.

It is a rare individual who will not have some response to these measures. However, if you cannot rekindle the lost flame of passion and desire, it's well to remember that libido normally has its own biorhythms and you may be in a temporary natural low. Take heart, for within the next few months your libido biorhythms may soar.

CHAPTER 12

FAREWELL MESSAGE

Millions of women suffer from hormonal imbalances from younger women traumatised by acne and premenstrual syndrome, to mothers struggling with postnatal depression, to grandmothers whose well deserved rest is broken by attacks of hot flushes. Hormonal upheavals can often be blamed for recurring headaches, sexual dysfunction, problems after hysterectomy and tubal ligation, unwanted hair, balding, chronic fatigue and general poor health. In the 1980s we discovered the vital link between oestrogen deficiency and the epidemic of osteoporosis and cardiovascular disease that cripples our ageing female population.

The majority of women have coped admirably with such hormonal problems, but in a significant minority these problems have had ruinous effects resulting in severe depression, family disruption, child battering, loss of self esteem, drug addiction and even suicide. It can be very frightening to feel a victim of one's hormones knowing that month after month unpleasant symptoms will recur to remind us of our uniquely female vulnerability.

When we understand that the hormonal system of a woman is such a delicate and complex network of interacting body chemicals, it is not surprising that at times it seems to go haywire! Not only are we vulnerable to our hormonal fluctuations, but our hormones are influenced by our weight, lifestyle, exercise patterns, stress, diet, nutritional imbalances and increasing age.

To fine-tune our hormones is obviously a very specialised and complicated endeavour. It is now possible for the first time in history to achieve this because of new breakthroughs in the speciality of women's hormones (Gynaecological Endocrinology).

Thankfully the attitude of society and doctors towards women with hormonal problems is changing. These problems have their hilarious side as depicted by the cartoons in this book, and they also have their tragic side with a propensity to devastate the lives of many women. Doctors are finally realising that women with hormonal problems want to be taken seriously and offered real and lasting solutions. They don't want to be stereotyped, patronised, trivialised or kept in the dark. It does not help to be told that your symptoms are inevitable, a natural part of womanhood or just a sign of your age.

I have written this book because every day I am challenged with women whose lives are being turned upside down by their hormones. These women are not neurotic or inadequate. They are intelligent, articulate, strong and very relatable personalities. They recognise that powerful hormonal forces are causing mental and/or physical changes that they need help to control so that their lives can be productive, fulfilled and stable.

I, myself, have had to find solutions for my own hormonally caused health problems that were preventing me from enjoying my life and "getting on with it", so to speak. Thus, I know how it feels to be a victim of one's hormones and thankfully I now know how to gain control over my own hormonal demons. To have overcome these horrible symptoms in myself and many of my patients has given me great satisfaction, understanding, compassion and relief.

I hope that this book enables me to share my many years of accumulated clinical research and experience with you. The book *Don't Let Your Hormones Ruin Your Life* aims to give you more insight into your mind and body and to show you all your treatment options with an emphasis on natural hormone and nutritional therapies. It is designed to give you all the tools that you will need to work with yourself and your doctor in conquering the many hormonal problems that may befall you.

GLOSSARY

ADRENAL GLANDS Two small glands sited on top of the kidneys which secrete steroid hormones and the stress hormone adrenalin.

AIDS Acquired Immune Deficiency Syndrome

ALOPECIA Abnormal and excessive loss of hair.

AMENORRHOEA An abnormal absence of menstrual bleeding.

AMINO ACIDS The building blocks of the body's protein. Ten of the amino acids are essential dietary components as they cannot be synthesised by the body. Dietary protein can only be considered first class if it contains all the 10 essential amino acids. First class protein can be obtained from animal and dairy products and also by combining any three of the following . . . nuts, grains, seeds, legumes at one meal.

AMPOULE A vial containing drugs or hormones for injection.

ANABOLIC STEROIDS Male hormones which stimulate the growth of bone and muscle.

ANDROGEN Male hormone

ANDROGENIC Having a masculine effect and thus stimulating growth of hair in a male pattern, oily skin, deepening of the voice and increased muscle mass.

ANGINA Chest pain caused by lack of blood supply to the heart.

ANTI-MALE HORMONE A hormone which blocks the synthesis and effects of male hormones and is capable of reversing masculine body features.

ANTIOXIDANT Substances such as vitamins A, C and E, beta-carotene and selenium which protect the cellular structures from oxidative damage caused by free radicals.

ATROPHY Wasting or thinning of tissues or organs.

BENIGN Non-cancerous or non-malignant

BIOFLAVONOIDS Bioflavonoids, sometimes referred to as vitamin P, are found in plants along with vitamin C and exert a beneficial effect upon the walls of the blood and lymphatic vessels. This is very helpful for women troubled with fluid retention and puffy limbs.

BODY MASS INDEX (B.M.I.) The B.M.I. is a scientific way of examining 'fatness' and 'thinness' and is worked out according to the formula B.M.I. = weight (kilogram) /height squared (metres^2). The normal B.M.I. ranges from 20 to 25 kg/m^2 and many hormonal and menstrual problems can be overcome by keeping weight in the normal B.M.I. range.

BODY TYPE There are four female body shapes or physiques, namely gynaeoid, thyroid, android and pituitary type. (See Page 109).

BREAKTHROUGH BLEEDING Irregular vaginal bleeding or spotting occurring in women when they are on the OCP or HRT.

CANCER A malignant growth/tumour with rapid multiplication of abnormal cells that may spread to and invade distant body parts.

CARDIOVASCULAR DISEASE Disease of the system of the blood circulation comprising the heart and blood vessels.

CAT SCAN A computerised X-ray of consecutive sections of the body

CELLULITE Fatty deposits resulting in a dimply or lumpy appearance of the skin which is difficult to remove with diet and exercise.

CERVIX The lower part of the uterus projecting down into the vagina. It is also called the mouth of the womb.

CHLAMYDIA A small bacteria which is a common cause of pelvic infection and infertility.

CHLOASMA Brownish pigmentation of the face caused by some types of hormones and pregnancy.

CHOLESTEROL A constituent of all animal fats and oils. It is found in the blood in two forms: 1. High Density Lipo-protein (HDL) which protects against atherosclerosis; 2. Low Density Lipo-protein (LDL) which promotes atherosclerosis.

CLITORIS The female equivalent of the penis. It is a small bulb found at the top of the vulva, just below the pubic bone and is covered by a hood of tissue. It contains erectile tissue which is very sensitive to stimulation and adds greatly to a woman's sexual response.

CLUSTER HEADACHE A severe and intense headache which lasts several hours, and may recur frequently over a six to eight week period.

COMBINED ORAL CONTRACEPTIVE PILL A contraceptive pill containing both female sex hormones, oestrogen and progesterone.

COMPLEX CARBOHYDRATES Carbohydrates occurring in an unprocessed form, and complexed with fibre, minerals and other nutrients. They are more slowly absorbed and utilised than processed or refined carbohydrates.

CONCEPTION The fertilisation of the female egg by the spermatozoa.

CONSENT FORM A legal document that you are required to sign, thereby giving your consent, before undergoing a surgical operation.

CONTRA-INDICATION A medical condition that makes it inadvisable to use a certain medication, eg. the presence of blood clots would contra-indicate the use of the contraceptive pill.

CORPUS LUTEUM The yellow coloured gland which is formed within the ovary from the remains of the follicle after it has released its contained egg at ovulation. The corpus luteum manufactures the hormone progesterone.

CORTISONE A steroid hormone made by the adrenal glands and also synthetically in laboratories. It improves well-being and has a powerful anti-inflammatory effect.

CUSHINGS SYNDROME   A collection of symptoms and signs such as a moon-shaped face, buffalo hump and high blood pressure caused by excessive amounts of cortisone.

CYSTIC ACNE   A skin disorder manifesting as blocked pores and pimples, many of which are blind cysts containing pus. It is a severe form of acne.

DIATHERMY   The surgical technique of burning tissues with a controlled electric current.

DIURETIC   A substance, whether synthetic or natural, which stimulates the kidneys to excrete salt (sodium chloride) and water, thereby relieving fluid retention.

ECTOPIC PREGNANCY   A pregnancy growing in an abnormal position, usually inside a fallopian tube.

ENDOCRINE GLANDS   Glands that manufacture and secrete hormones.

ENDOCRINOLOGIST   A medical specialist in diseases of the endocrine glands and their hormones.

ENDOCRINOLOGY   The study and treatment of disorders of the glands and the hormones they secrete.

ENDOMETRIOSIS   The presence of endometrium (which is normally confined inside the uterine cavity) outside of the uterus scattered about inside the abdomen and pelvic cavities.

ENZYMES   Proteins produced by living cells which function as catalysts in specific biochemical reactions.

ESSENTIAL FATTY ACIDS   Fatty acids necessary for cellular metabolism which cannot be made by the body, but must be supplied in the diet. Suitable sources are oil of evening primrose, fish, fish oil, nuts, seeds and their oils.

EVENING PRIMROSE OIL   The oil extracted from the beautiful evening primrose plant which is renowned for its healing and tonifying properties. It is an excellent source of the omega 6 fatty acids, in particular the essential fatty acid known as gamma linolenic acid (GLA).

FALLOPIAN TUBES   The tubes which carry the egg (ovum) from the ovary to the uterus. Fertilisation of the egg occurs in the outer part of the fallopian tube.

FEMALE SEX HORMONES   The two sex hormones produced by the female ovary — namely oestrogen and progesterone.

FERTILISATION   The union of the female egg (ovum) with the male egg (spermatozoa) which occurs in the fallopian tube.

FIBROIDS   Non-cancerous growths of the uterus consisting of muscle and fibrous tissue.

FOETUS   A developing human from the end of the eighth week of pregnancy up until birth.

FOLLICLE STIMULATING HORMONE (FSH) A hormone secreted by the pituitary gland which reaches the ovaries via the blood circulation and stimulates the growth of ovarian follicles (eggs).

'FRIENDLY PROGESTERONES' Those types of progesterone that exert a favourable effect upon our blood vessels and skin and do not increase cholesterol, promote weight gain or masculine changes in the skin. Examples are cyproterone acetate, gestodene or desogestrel.

FRIGID (SEXUAL) Sexually unresponsive and disinterested.

GALACTORRHOEA The presence of milk or milky fluid in the breasts when not breast-feeding.

GAMMA LINOLENIC ACID (GLA) An omega 6 essential fatty acid that is used to synthesise prostaglandins. It has an anti-inflammatory effect in the body. Good sources of GLA are breast milk, oil of evening primrose, oil from the borage plant and blackcurrant seed oil.

GLANDS Organs or tissues, generally soft and fleshy in consistency, that manufacture and secrete or excrete hormones that exert their effect elsewhere in the body.

GYNAECOLOGY Study of diseases of women.

GYNAECOLOGICAL ENDOCRINOLOGY Study of the hormones produced by women. It is a relatively new medical specialty which is expanding rapidly and brings the promise of exciting new developments and hope for many women.

HIRSUTISM A condition of excessive facial and body hair, excluding the scalp.

HORMONES Chemicals produced by various glands which are then transported around the body.

HORMONE REPLACEMENT THERAPY (HRT) The administration of hormonal preparations (natural or synthetic) to replace the loss of natural hormones produced by various glands.

HYPOTHALAMUS A major control centre situated at the base of the brain, regulating body temperature, thirst, appetite and other hormonal glands. It releases hormones that travel directly to the pituitary gland via a stalk.

HYSTERECTOMY Surgical removal of the uterus.

IMMUNE SYSTEM The defence and surveillance system of the body which protects against infection by micro-organisms and invasion by foreign proteins.

IMPLANT A chemical substance, hormone or object, that is surgically implanted into a part of the body.

INFLAMMATION A condition characterised by swelling, redness, heat and pain in any tissue as a result of trauma, irritation, infection or imbalances in immune function.

LAPAROSCOPE   A long thin telescopic instrument utilising a fiberoptic lighting system, that is inserted through a half inch incision in the abdominal wall. It functions like a hollow flashlight enabling the surgeon to view internal organs and insert operating instruments through its hollow bore.

LIBIDO   Level of sexual desire.

LUTEINISING HORMONE (LH)   A hormone produced by the pituitary gland which acts on the ovary to cause ovulation and the production of progesterone.

MALE HORMONE   A hormone which promotes masculine characteristics in the body such as facial and body hair, balding, acne, deepening of the voice and increased libido.

MALIGNANT   Cancerous.

MANIC DEPRESSION   A mental illness characterised by episodes of euphoric and delusional hyperactivity alternating with deep depressions.

MENOPAUSE   The final cessation of menstruation. The last period.

MENSTRUAL CLOCK   A specialised part of the hypothalamus regulating the cyclical timing of menstrual bleeding.

MENSTRUAL CYCLE   The period of time from the first day of menstruation to the first day of the next menstruation.

MENSTRUATION   Monthly bleeding from the vagina in women of child bearing age, caused by shedding of the lining of the womb.

METABOLIC RATE   The rate at which the body converts food energy into kinetic energy.

METABOLISM   Chemical processes utilising the raw materials of nutrients, oxygen and vitamins along with enzymes to produce energy for bodily functions.

MICROSURGICAL TECHNIQUES   Surgery performed on small parts of the body such as nerve fibres, blood vessels or fallopian tubes, requiring the use of the operating microscope.

NATUROPATHIC MEDICINE   The treatment of illness with naturally occurring substances such as organic foods, juices, nutritional supplements and herbs.

NEURO-TRANSMITTERS   Chemicals and hormones that transmit messages between the cells and nervous pathways of the brain.

NON-ANDROGENIC   Not causing masculine effects in the body.

OESTRADIOL   A natural oestrogen made by the ovaries. It is the most potent of all the natural oestrogens.

OESTROGENS   The female sex hormones secrete by the ovary being responsible for the female charateristics of breasts, feminine curves and menstruation.

ORAL   Denoting a drug to be taken by mouth.

ORGASM   The physical and emotional culmination of the sexual act.

OSTEOPOROSIS Loss of bone mass due to loss of bone minerals. Skeletal atrophy. Porous condition of bones.

OVARIAN BLOOD SUPPLY The blood carried to the ovaries via the ovarian arteries which branch off from the uterine blood vessels. The ovarian arteries run alongside the fallopian tubes.

OVARIES The female sex glands (gonads) located on each side of the uterus which produce eggs and the female sex hormones (oestrogen and progesterone).

OVULATION The release of the egg from the ovary occurring around mid-cycle.

OVULATION PAIN Pain occuring at ovulation which may be sharp and severe and last from a few minutes up to 12 hours.

PARENTERAL Taken into the body or adminstered in a manner other than by mouth or the digestive canal.

PELVIC INFLAMMATORY DISEASE (PID) Inflammation of the pelvic organs, particularly the uterus and fallopian tubes, caused by infectious micro-organisms.

PESSARY An oval shaped suppository containing drugs or hormones designed to be inserted into the vagina.

PHYSIOLOGICAL Consistent with the normal functioning of an organism.

PITUITARY GLAND A mushroom-shaped gland connected by a vascular stalk to the base of the brain. The pituitary gland manufactures hormones which in turn control other hormonal glands, such as the thyroid, adrenals, ovaries, testicles and breasts.

PLACENTA The hormonal organ formed in the lining of the uterus by the union of the uterine mucous membrane with the membranes of the foetus to provide for the nourishment of the foetus and the elimination of its waste products.

POLYCYSTIC OVARIAN SYNDROME A condition of hormonal imbalance characterised by excessive male hormones and irregular menstruation. It is strongly inherited and may be triggered by stress or weight gain.

POLYCYSTIC OVARIES The type of ovaries present in women with the Polycystic Ovarian Syndrome. They have more than 10 small follicles per ovary aligned around the edge of the ovary, whereas in a 'normal' ovary they are distributed more evenly throughout the ovary. They can be seen by an ultrasound scan of the pelvis.

POMEROY TECHNIQUE OF TUBAL LIGATION In this method the gynaecologist lifts each fallopian tube to create a loop, ties the base of the loop tightly together with a suture, and cuts off the top of the loop. The suture is gradually absorbed and the two scarred ends of the tube pull apart, leaving a gap between them.

POST-MENOPAUSE The period of time after the menopause.

POSTNATAL After childbirth.

POST-PARTUM After childbirth.

PREMATURE MENOPAUSE If menopause occurs before the age of 40, it is considered as premature.

PRE-MENOPAUSAL The years, generally 4 to 5, leading up to the menopause, characterised by a time of hormonal imbalance.

PREMENSTRUAL SYNDROME A collection of variable symptoms such as mood disturbance, headaches, abdominal bloating etc., recurring on a cyclical basis in the one to two weeks, leading up to menstrual bleeding.

PROGESTOGENS Synthetic forms of the natural female hormone progesterone. They are commonly used in the OCP and HRT and regulate menstrual bleeding. Examples are norethisterone, norgestrel and medroxy-progesterone acetate.

PROGESTERONE ONLY PILL A contraceptive pill containing only one hormone, namely a progestogen such as norethisterone. It is also known as the mini pill.

PROLACTIN A hormone secreted by the pituitary gland that stimulates milk production in the breasts.

PROSTAGLANDINS Chemicals manufactured throughout the body which exert a hormone-like effect and influence muscular contraction, circulation and inflammation.

PROSTATE GLAND This gland is located just below the bladder in men and secretes fluid when the ejaculation of semen is imminent.

PSYCHOSIS A severe mental disorder characterised by delusions, hallucinations, confusion, and a breakdown of reality.

PSYCHOSOMATIC Physical symptoms that are due to psychological and emotional causes and not due to physical disease.

PSYCHOTHERAPY The treatment of mental and emotional imbalance through analysis of the thought processes, defence mechanisms and subconscious mind.

PSYCHOTIC A mental illness or patient having the features of a psychosis.

PSYCHOTROPIC DRUGS Drugs that act primarily on the brain. Examples are sedatives, tranquillisers and anti-depressants.

PUERPERIUM The period of time after childbirth required to return the genital organs to their pre-pregnant size and condition. This takes six to eight weeks.

SCAN/ULTRASOUND See ultrasound

SEBACEOUS GLANDS These are the tiny oil producing glands in the skin. If they over-produce oil and/or become obstructed, pimples or acne will result.

SEROTONIN A potent brain chemical which regulates sleep, mood, libido and appetite.

SEX HORMONES The male and female hormones produced by the testicles, ovaries, adrenal glands and fat eg. oestrogen, testosterone and progesterone.

STEROID DRUGS AND HORMONES This group of hormones have a ring-like chemical structure. Examples of steroid hormones are cortisone and the male and female sex hormones.

STROKE   Brain damage resulting from a disturbance of blood supply to the brain.

SYMPATHETIC NERVOUS SYSTEM   That part of the autonomic (automatic) nervous system which prepares the body for stress by raising the blood pressure and pulse rate via the release of stress hormones.

SYMPTOMS   Physical complaints.

SYNDROME   A group of signs and symptoms that collectively characterise a disease.

SYNERGISTIC NUTRIENT   A nutrient which helps or increases the effect of other body nutrients.

TAILOR-MADE ORAL CONTRACEPTIVE PILL   A pill that is specially designed for you by your doctor to suit your unique physical, mental and contraceptive needs.

TESTOSTERONE   The major male sex hormone.

THYROID GLAND   The endocrine gland situated in front of the neck which produces the hormone thyroxine.

TRIGLYCERIDES   One of the blood fats, the level of which is influenced by diet, alcohol, exercise and drugs.

TUBAL LIGATION   The surgical obstruction or interruption of the fallopian tubes for the purpose of permanent sterilization.

TUMOUR   An abnormal growth which may be cancerous or benign.

UTERUS   The womb.

UROLOGIST   A doctor who specialises in diseases of the kidneys and urinary tract.

ULTRASOUND SCAN   A method of visualising the internal organs, foetus and blood vessels. Ultrasound does not incur any radiation exposure and utilises very high frequency sound waves (more than 20,000 hertz) that are above the audible limit.

VAGINA   The genital canal or passage leading from the uterus to the vulva; it accommodates the penis during intercourse.

VAGINAL DIAPHRAGM   A soft rubber cap that fits snugly over the cervix and is used for contraception.

VASOACTIVE DRUGS   Drugs acting on the blood vessels.

VIRILIZATION   The development of masculine physical characteristics.

VULVA   Female external genitalia. Also known as the lips of the vaginal opening.

APPENDIX — PRODUCT AVAILABILITY CHART

MEDICATION	AUSTRALIA	NZ	USA	UK
PROGESTERONE				
NATURAL				
Vaginal pessaries/suppositories	progesterone		progesterone	Cyclogest
Tablets/Lozenges		may need to import	natural progesterone	natural progesterone
Injections	Proluton 25 mg	Gestone 25-100mg	Progesterone	Gestone 25-100mg
SEMI-NATURAL				
Tablets	Duphaston	Duphaston	unavailable	Duphaston
Injections	Proluton Depot	Proluton Depot	unavailable	Proluton Depot
SYNTHETIC				
Tablets	Primolut/Provera	Primolut/Provera	Norlutate/Provera	Primolut/Provera
OESTROGENS				
NATURAL				
Oestradiol Tablets	Progynova	Progynova	Estrace	Progynova
Patches	Estraderm	Estraderm	Estraderm	Estraderm
Injections	Primogyn Depot	Benztrone	need to import	need to import
Vaginal cream	Dienoestrol	Dienoestrol	Estrace	Dienoestrol
Vaginal pessaries	Kolpon	Kolpon	Ogen	Vagifem
Oestrogen & Testosterone Injections	Primodian Depot	unavailable	unavailable	unavailable
SYNTHETIC				
Ethinyloestradiol Tablets	Estigyn	Ethinyloestradiol	Estinyl	Ethinyloestradiol
MALE HORMONES				
Testosterone Injections	Sustanon/Primoteston Depot	Sustanon/Primoteston Depot	Depot — Testosterone	Sustanon/Primoteston Depot
Testosterone Tablets	Testomet/Andriol	Testomet/Andriol	Android	Restandol
ORAL CONTRACEPTIVE PILLS (OCPs)				
FEMININE				
Ethinyloestradiol + desogestrel	Marvelon, Triodene	Marvelon/Mercilon	unavailable	Marvelon/Mercilon
Ethinyloestradiol + cyproterone acetate	Diane	Diane	unavailable	Diane
Ethinyloestradiol + gestodene	Femodene	Femodene	unavailable	Femodene

TRIPHASIC LOW DOSE Ethinyloestradiol + levonorgestrel	TriQuilar/Triphasil	TriQuilar/Triphasil	Triquilar/Triphasil	Triphasil/Tri-levlen	Logynon/Trinordiol
PROGESTERONE ONLY PILLS					
Levonorgestrel	Microlut	Microlut	Microlut	Ovrette	Microval
Norethisterone	Noriday	Noriday	Noriday	Micronor	Noriday
ANTI-MALE HORMONES					
cyproterone acetate	Androcur	Androcur	Androcur	unavailable	Androcur
spironolactone	Aldactone	Aldactone	Aldactone	Aldactone	Aldactone
THYROID HORMONES					
T3 Liothyronine/T4 Thyroxine	Tertroxin/Oroxine	Tertroxin/Oroxine	Tertroxin/Eltroxin	Cytomel/Levoxine	Tertroxin/Thyroxine
DIURETICS					
Potassium Sparing	Moduretic	Moduretic	Moduretic	Moduretic	Moduretic
DRUGS WITH HORMONE ACTION					
Bromocriptine	Parlodel	Parlodel	Parlodel	Parlodel	Parlodel
ANTI-DEPRESSANTS					
Monoamine Oxidase Inhibitors	Parnate/Nardil/aurorix	Parnate/Nardil	Parnate/Nardil	Parnate/Nardil	Parnate/Nardil
Tricyclics	Tofranol/Sinequan/Prothiaden	Imipramin/Sinequan/Prothiaden	Tofranil/Sinequan/Prothiaden	Tofranil/Sinequan	Tofranil/Sinequan/Prothiaden
MIGRAINE					
Ergotamine for pain	Cafergot	Cafergot	Cafergot	Cafergot	Cafergot
Maxalon for nausea	Maxalon	Maxalon	Maxalon	Reglan	Maxalon
ACNE					
CREAMS & LOTIONS					
Retinoic acid – also anti-ageing	Retin A cream	Retin A cream	Retin A cream	Retin A cream	Retin A cream
Anti-inflammatory	Neomedrol lotion	Neomedrol lotion	Neomedrol lotion	Neodecadron cream	Neomedrone cream
TABLETS					
Isotretinoin	Roaccutane	Roaccutane	Roaccutane	Accutane	Roaccutane

AVAILABILITY OF NATURAL PROGESTERONE

Australia — Stenlake Chemist, 169 Oxford Street, Bondi Junction. (02) 9387 3205

USA — Better Health & Medical Group Inc., 1491 E. LaPalma Ave., Suite No. C. Anaheim, CA 92805. Phone: (714) 774 7490. Fax: (714) 774 2826
Approximate cost — 50 suppositories/pessaries (400mg strength) — costs $56.25
St. Mark Medical Group, 7648 Seville Ave., Huntington Park CA 90255. Phone: (213) 587 1175

UK — The Doctors Laboratory, 58 Wimpole St. London WIM-7DE. Phone: (01) 224 1001. Fax: (01) 224 0341.
Approximate cost — 40 ampoules of progesterone (strength 100mg) — costs £38.28p.

INDEX

HELPFUL ORGANISATIONS FOR WOMEN

If you wish to receive information from the following organisations, always send a stamped self-addressed envelope along with your request.

AUSTRALIA

NEW SOUTH WALES

Women's Health Advisory Service (WHAS), 155 Eagle Creek Rd, Werombi 2570, Phone (046) 531 445.

Menopause Clinic, Royal Hospital for Women, 188 Oxford Street, Paddington 2021. Phone: (02) 339 4111.

Menopause & PMS Support Group, 155 Eagle Creek Rd, Werombi 2570, They offer counselling and nutritional advice and a mail order service for women's health vitamins, nutritional supplements and cosmetics. Phone (046) 531 445 Fax (046) 531 144.

Women's Health, Information, Resource & Crisis Centre (WHIRCCA), PO Box 507, Leichhardt 2040. Phone: (02) 550 9609.

Australian Family Planning Association, 161 Broadway, Sydney 2007. Phone: (02) 211 0244. Branches in every state.

VICTORIA

Key Centre for Women's Health in Society, University of Melbourne, 209 Graham Street, Carlton 3053. Phone: (03) 344 4333.

Victorian Endometriosis Association. Phone: (03) 879 1289.

Aboriginal Health Service. Phone: (03) 419 3000.

QUEENSLAND

The Women's Health Centre — Brisbane, 165 Gregory Terrace, Spring Hill. PO Box 665 Spring Hill 4004. Phone: (07) 839 9988 or 008 017 676 toll free.

WESTERN AUSTRALIA

Menopause Clinic, King Edward Memorial Hospital for Women, Bagot Road, Subiaco. Phone: (09) 340 1355.

Women's Health Care Association Inc., 92 Thomas Street, West Perth 6005. Phone: (09) 321 2833.

Women's Multicultural Health Centre. Phone: (09) 335 8214.

Family Planning Association. Phone: (09) 227 6177.

SOUTH AUSTRALIA
Menopause Clinic, Queen Victoria Hospital, 160 Fullarton Road, Rose Park. Phone: (08) 332 4888.

NORTHERN TERRITORY
Menopause Clinic, Family Planning Association, Shop 11, Rapid Creek Shopping Centre, Rapid Creek. Phone: (089) 48 0144.

TASMANIA
Family Planning Association, 73 Federal Street, North Hobart. Phone: (002) 34 7200.

Hobart Women's Health Centre, 9 Pierce Street, Moonah. Phone: (002) 28 0997.

NEW ZEALAND
National Council of Women of New Zealand, PO Box 12117, Wellington North.

UNITED KINGDOM
British Pregnancy Advisory Service, Austy Manor, Wootton Wawen Solihull, West Midlands B956BX. Phone: (05) 642 3225.

Women's Health and Reproductive Rights Information Centre (WHRRIC), 52 Featherstone Street, London ECI 8RT. Phone: (071) 251 6332 or 251 6580.

Women and Medical Practice (WAMP), 666 High Road, Tottenham, London N17. Phone: (081) 885 2277.

Women's Nutritional Advisory Service and PMT Advisory Service, PO Box 268, Hove, East Sussex BN3 6RH. Phone: (027) 377 1366.

National Osteoporosis Society, Barton Meade House, PO Box 10, Radstock, Bath BA3 3YB. Phone: (07) 613 2472.

Healthwise, 27-35 Mortimer Street, London WIN 7RJ.

Hysterectomy Support Group, Rivendell, Warren Way Lower Heswall Wirral Merseyside. Phone: (051) 342 3167 or London Group, 11 Henryson Road, Brockley, London SE4 1HL. Phone: (01) 690 5987.

UNITED STATES OF AMERICA
Endometriosis Association, PO Box 92187, Milwaukee, WI 53202. Phone: (414) 962 8972.

Institute for Reproductive Health, 8721 Beverley Boulevard, Los Angeles, CA 90048. Phone: (213) 854 7714.

The Resource Centre, American College of Obstetricians and Gynaecologists, 600 Maryland Avenue SW Washington DC 20024-2588. Phone: (202) 863 2518.

American Fertility Society, 2131 Magnolia Avenue, Birmingham, AL 35256. Phone: (205) 251 9764.

American Cancer Society, 777 Third Avenue, New York NY 10017. Phone: (212) 586 8700. Consult local branches in major cities.

American Association of Sex Educators, Counsellors and Therapists, 11 Dupont Circle NW Washington DC 20036. Phone: (202) 462 1171.

National Women's Network, 244 Seventh Street SE Washington DC 20003.

Premenstrual Syndrome Access, PO Box 9326, Madison, WI 53715. Phone: (800) 237 4666. or (800) 558 7046.

Women's Association for Research in Menopause, 128 E 56th Street, New York NY 10022.

CANADA

Women's Health Education Network, PO Box 1276, Truro, Nova Scotia B2N5N2.

THE BODY SHAPING DIET

Each Body Type—Android, Gynaeoid, Lymphatic and Thyroid has a different hormonal balance and metabolism and because of this is prone to weight gain in different areas of the body.

To lose weight efficiently and permanently, and to get back your body shape you must follow a diet that gives you the correct food combinations to match your body type. This diet is called The Body Shaping Diet and enables you to control your weight easily by balancing your hormones and stimulating your metabolism. For full details refer to my new book *The Body Shaping Diet*, published by the Womens Health Advisory Service (see back of this book for details on how to order).

WOMEN'S HEALTH ADVISORY NETWORK

155 Eagle Creek Road Werombi NSW 2570
Phone: (046) 531445   Fax: (046) 531144

Do you want to stay in touch with the latest advances in menopause, hormone replacement therapy, anti-ageing techniques, breast care. skin care, nutrition, naturopathic medicine, hormonal problems, improving your sex drive, candida, weight control, body shaping, where to find the best medical specialists and other health issues of vital concem to women?

You can do this by joining our network. This will keep you in touch and give you access to all these things through our newsletter.

Network members receive our exciting newsletter called "What's News", published and mailed to you every 8 weeks. The newsletter contains feature articles on women's health by **Dr. Sandra Cabot** MBBS, DRCOG, **Dr. Oscar Honky**, specialist obstetrician and gynaecologist, **Dr. Lawrence Ho**, plastic surgeon, **Bianca Bozlc**, beautician and industrial chemist, **Florence Thomas**, counsellor and social welfare worker, **Trixie Whitmore**, environmental consultant.

We will include topics of interest for the whole family from this impressive team of professionals.

Being a health network member puts you in touch with a network of "switched on", inspirational and helpful health care workers.

• *If you are concemed that chemicals and toxins are making you sick,* Trixie Whitmore can help you—write to P.O. Box 266 Pymble 2073 and look for her regular newsletter articles.

• *If you are not coping with stress or depression,* Florence Thomas or Ricki Hilder can help you—call Florence on (02) 9398 9448—Box 4, 55B Frenchmans Rd Randwick 2031 or call Ricki on (02) 9399 9820.

• *If you want to stay fit and firm,* contact Ann Mader, our specialist on women's exercise on (02) 9909 3524 or write to Unit 6, 50-52 Earle Street, Cremorne 2090.

• *Do you want to receive the highest quality natural* vitamins, evening primrose oil, skin care products and health books, mailed to you at discount prices?

IF SO, JOIN OUR NETWORK!

You can Join our Network for 12 months and have all these benefits for only $55.00.

✄ _____

HOW TO JOIN THE WOMEN'S HEALTH ADVISORY NETWORK.

Send $55 to Women's Health Advisory Service (WHAS) with your details and you will be entered on our Computer Mailing List and receive a Membership Card and number, your first Newsletter, a Naturopathic Table and 1 FREE copy of Dr Sandra Cabot's booklet called "The Handbag Health Guide". Send your $55 to WHAS, 155 Eagle Creek Road, Werombi 2570.1f you have a Credit Card (VISA, Mastercard or Bankcard), you can phone us on (046) 53 1445 or fax us on (046) 53 1144 with your details.

YOUR NAME ....

YOUR ADDRESS...

....POSTCODE ....YOUR PHONE..............................

Send Cheque/Money Order for: $55.00 to WHAS or DEBIT my Credit Card ....

VISA ☐ MASTERCARD ☐ BANKCARD ☐

YOUR CREDIT CARD NO. ....CARD EXPIRY DATE.................

Your Signature...

BODY SHAPING CLINIC

BODY SHAPING STRATEGIES

The links between your Body Type, hormones and body weight are important and explain the fact that the same diet does not work equally well for all women. There are four basic Body Types—namely Android, Gynaeoid, Lymphatic and Thyroid (see diagram) and each type has distinct hormonal and metabolic characteristics. In other words we have biochemical individuality that needs to be taken into account when designing an eating plan to normalise weight. The Body Shaping Diet has been designed to stimulate the metabolic rate and promote hormonal balance in each of the body types. This will enable efficient and lasting weight loss to occur from the areas where hormonally dependent fat excess has occurred. So by understanding the vital links between your body type and the areas where you accumulate hormonally dependant excess fat you have the tools to lose weight from where you so desire.

For all women with excess weight and underactive metabolism it is vital to treat the LYMPHATIC SYSTEM (see diagram lymphatic system). The Body Shaping Diet is a cleansing diet and works on the lymphatic system thus reducing fluid retention, mucous congestion and cellulite. Our body shaping counsellors can help you to understand the lymphatic system and its importance in weight loss and well being.

Many women need help in maintaining a healthy weight because they are very confused as to the finer details of food combining and the ratio of fat/protein carbohydrates suitable for their individual metabolism. This is explained in the book called the "BODY SHAPING DIET" written by Dr Sandra Cabot which provides delicious and easily prepared meals to suit your Body Type.

Some women also find it difficult to determine their Body Type especially if they have become very overweight and need a trained Body Shaping counsellor to help them. These counsellors are able to tell you what Body Type you are and therefore which diet suits you best. They can also provide lymphatic massage with Svelte Body Contour Cream for those with cellulite and fluid retention.

Our counsellors can monitor your progress and keep you inspired when your self esteem and will power are flagging. They can advise you on natural foods and supplements to aid your metabolism which makes weight loss quicker.

Our Body Shaping counsellors are trained by Sandra Cabot.

If you would like to speak with one of our Body Shaping counsellors or our naturopath call us today on

       046-531445
  or 018-420010
  or 02-4565052
  or 02-6651627
  or 015-100920
  or 02-3316932

Body Types

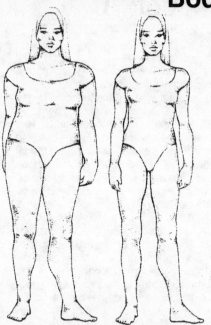

*Android body shape (left) overweight,
(right) ideal weight*

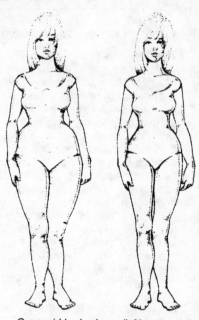

*Gynacoid body shape (left) overweight,
(right) ideal weight*

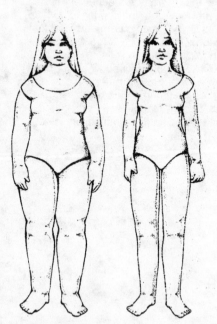

*Lymphatic body shape (left) overweight,
(right) ideal weight*

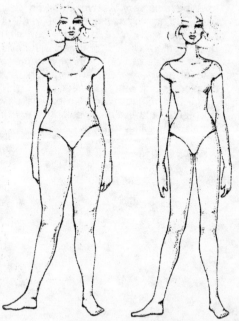

*Thyroid body shape (left) overweight,
(right) ideal weight*

The Lymphatic System

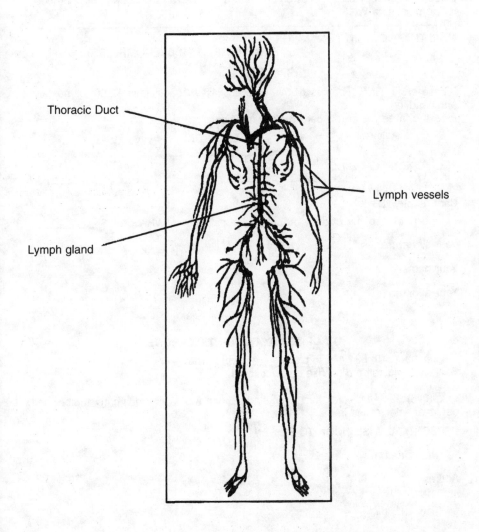

Thoracic Duct

Lymph vessels

Lymph gland

DON'T LET YOUR HORMONES RUIN YOUR LIFE

GIFT SUGGESTION FROM THE WOMEN'S HEALTH ADVISORY SERVICE

If you would like to send/receive GIFT COPIES of this book, personally autographed by the author, to a friend or relative simply fill in this coupon and return it to the WHAS with your payment. The WHAS will then either post it to you or direct to the person you specify on the coupon below. You may cut off the coupon or photocopy it and post it to WHAS.

MAIL THIS COUPON TO: WHAS
155 EAGLE CREEK RD, WEROMBI 2570
AUSTRALIA

Please send _____ copies of this book at $15.95 each, plus $2.00 for postage and handling.

Please charge my credit card (tick correct card):

BANKCARD☐   MASTERCARD☐   VISA☐

YOUR CREDIT CARD NO: ☐☐☐☐☐☐☐☐☐☐☐☐☐☐☐☐☐☐☐☐

Card Expiry Date. . . . .

or find enclosed my cheque/money order payable to WHAS for $_____

Your signature . . . .

Your name . . . .

Your address . . . .

. . . . P/C . . . . Your telephone no . . . .

OR ORDER BY FAX OR TELEPHONE

Telephone: (046) 531 445 to place a credit card order —
Bankcard, Mastercard or Visa only accepted.

Fax: (046) 531 144 — fax this completed coupon with your credit card number and personal details filled in.

PERSON YOU WISH BOOK TO BE SENT TO:

To whom (name) . . . .

Address . . . .

. . . . P/C . . . .

Please fill in all parts of this coupon, including post codes, and check your credit card number and expiry date before signing. Prompt delivery is assured.

MENOPAUSE – YOU CAN GIVE IT A MISS!

Doctor Sandra Cabot's book *Menopause — You Can Give It A Miss!* can be sent to you or a friend with our mail order system. This book describes all the powerful tools available to enable you to avoid the negative aspects and fears of the menopause. Dr Cabot describes the use of natural hormone replacement therapy, 'designer HRT', essential tests and a naturopathic anti-ageing plan. Subjects discussed are ■ What causes the menopause? ■ How do you know if your body lacks oestrogen? ■ A plan to avoid osteoporosis ■ Diet and exercise ■ How to maintain your sexuality and libido ■ Natural hormone tablets, injections, patches, creams, implants ■ Strategies to overcome side effects from HRT ■ Premature menopause ■ Nutritional supplements to help with menopause and ageing. ■ Alternatives to Hormone Replacement Therapy.

TO ORDER THE MENOPAUSE BOOK MAIL THIS COUPON TO:

WHAS
155 EAGLE CREEK RD, WEROMBI 2570
AUSTRALIA

Or order by PHONE (046) 531 445
or FAX (046) 531 144 using this completed coupon. You need a valid credit card to order by phone or fax.

Please rush me_____ copies of the Menopause Book at $15.95 each plus $2.00 for postage and handling.

Charge my credit card (tick correct card):

      BANKCARD☐   MASTERCARD☐   VISA☐

YOUR CREDIT CARD NO: ☐☐☐☐☐☐☐☐☐☐☐☐☐☐☐☐

Card Expiry Date. . . . .

OR find enclosed my cheque/money order payable to WHAS for $_____

Your name . . . .

Your address . . . .

P/C . . . . Your signature . . . .

Only Bankcard, Mastercard or Visa is accepted. Please fill in all parts of this coupon, including post code, credit card number and expiry date before signing.

THE BODY SHAPING DIET

Do you diet and lose weight in the wrong places?
Do you wish to improve your body shape?
Is your cellulite out of control?
Are you getting fat but don't know why?
Are you looking for an easy, safe, economical and nutritious diet?
If so, the *Body Shaping Diet* is for you!

There are four different body types—ANDROID, GYNAEOID, LYMPHATIC and THYROID—each has distinct hormonal and metabolic differences. To lose weight efficiently and get back your body shape you must follow a diet that has correct food combinations to match YOUR body type. This is called The Body Shaping Diet.

To order *The Body Shaping Diet* mail this coupon to:

WHAS
155 EAGLE CREEK RD, WEROMBI 2570
AUSTRALIA

Or order by PHONE (046) 531 445
or FAX (046) 531 144 using this completed coupon. You need a valid credit card to order by phone or fax.

Please rush me _____ copies of The Body Shaping Diet Book at $16.95 each plus $2.00 for postage and handling.

Card my credit card (tick correct card):

　　　　BANKCARD ☐　　　　MASTERCARD ☐　　　　VISA ☐

YOUR CREDIT CARD NO: ☐☐☐☐☐☐☐☐☐☐☐☐☐☐☐☐

Card Expiry Date ....

OR find enclosed my cheque/money order payable to WHAS for $

Your name ....

Your address ....

P/C .... Your signature ....

Only Bankcard, Mastercard or Visa is accepted. Please fill in all parts of this coupon, including post code, credit card number and expiry date before signing.